VETERINARIANS, HUMANE SOCIETIES, AND OTHERS AGAINST ANIMALS

VETERINARIANS, HUMANE SOCIETIES, AND OTHERS AGAINST ANIMALS

The Politics Behind the Killing of America's Pets

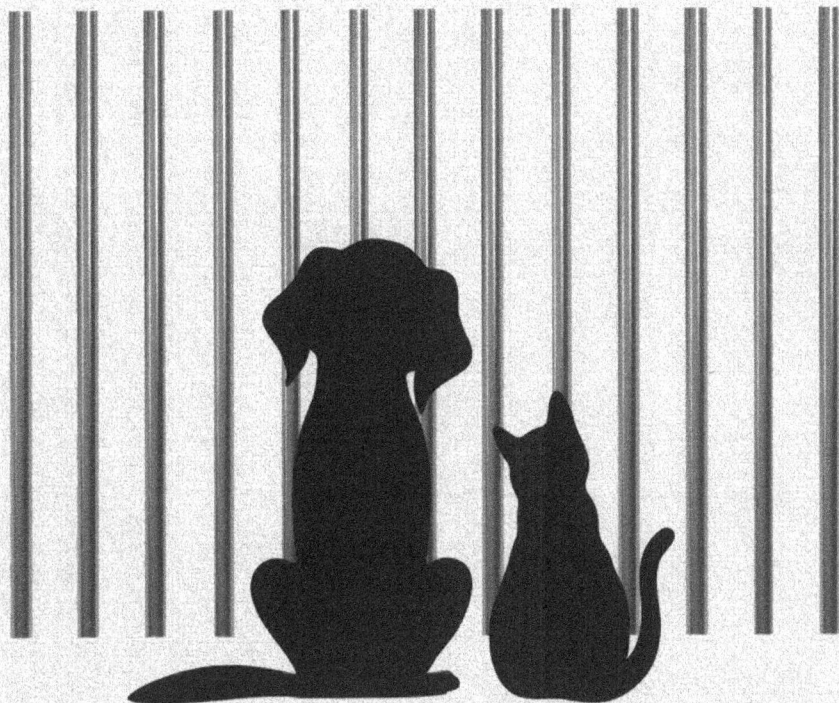

DELORIS DELLUOMO

Bink Books
Bedazzled Ink Publishing Company • Fairfield, California

paperback 978-1-949290-25-7

Cover Design
by

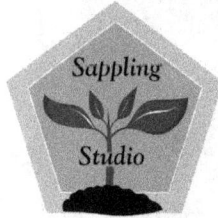

Bink Books
a division of
Bedazzled Ink Publishing, LLC
Fairfield, California
http://www.bedazzledink.com

For Dan and Dana . . .

. . . and all the loving and beautiful animals that have passed through my life, leaving their memories burned indelibly into my psyche and taking with them, each and every one, a part of my heart and soul.

ACKNOWLEDGMENTS

Oddly enough, considering the unique title of this book, my first expression of appreciation is to the veterinarians all across this country who have risked the wrath of their Boards, as well as their careers, to perform life-saving, high-volume, low-cost neuters and spays, whether or not it is within their own clinics or for non-profit neuter/spay programs. While the most vocal opponents of our work here in Oklahoma have been veterinarians and the Oklahoma State Board of Veterinary Medical Examiners, the irony is that without veterinarians, we would never have been able to operate a successful neuter/spay clinic for the past thirty-five years.

Dr. Jeff Tidwell of Marlow, Oklahoma, was the first veterinarian to step out on a limb and, at least for a short period of time, help us get the Animal Birth Control Clinic up and going, staying with us until his license was threatened by the OSBVME. We will always be grateful to Dr. Tidwell.

Local veterinarian Dr. Larry Chambers spent a short time with the clinic until his license was threatened by the OSBVME.

Dr. Becky Brewer-Walker, a relief veterinarian from Chickasha, Oklahoma, saved the day for us and came on one day's notice, with twenty dogs and cats in kennels awaiting surgery, at a time when the previous veterinarian had walked out due to pressure from the OSBVME. At the time, she was providing euthanasia services for the city shelter in her community and understood the critical need for neutering and spaying. She is a credit to the profession.

Dr. Zbigniew Richard Zdunek managed to hang on for approximately eighteen months before he was forced by the Board to leave. We sincerely thank Dr. Zdunek for his services and his belief in what we were doing.

Dr. Kenneth Reynolds, who ultimately performed surgeries at the Animal Birth Control Clinic for 20 years, not without unrelenting harassment from the Board, but due to a Federal Trade Commission ruling in the clinic's favor. Dr. Reynolds remains with the Clinic to this day on off-surgery days to administer vaccinations. Whatever other local veterinarians had to say about Dr. Reynolds, they could never find a reason to fault his immaculate surgical skills.

The late Dr. William Barrett drove to Lawton from Texas and, in order to be available for any unforeseen emergency, spent the night in what was once a kennel that housed twenty-eight rescued bird dogs and had been turned into a small apartment right beside the clinic. We will always be grateful to Dr. Barrett.

Dr. Kevin Rouillard drives from nearby Wichita Falls, Texas, and currently performs anywhere from seventy-five to a hundred surgeries in just two days at the clinic. We thank him for his dedication and his immaculate surgical skills.

This list of veterinarians would not be complete without recognizing one of the most talented veterinarians in the high-volume neuter/spay arena, the late Dr. Terry Yunker, who helped out when Lawton enacted the BAT (Breeding, Advertising, Transfer) law and there were more animals needing to be neutered and spayed than one veterinarian could handle. Dr. Yunker spent many years of his life on Indian reservations making sure every dog and cat in sight was "fixed." His love for animals and his knowledge of the need for neutering and spaying in the battle against pet overpopulation will not soon be forgotten.

There can be no doubt about the contributions humane societies have made to the cause of animal welfare. Tens of thousands of well-meaning individuals who make up the humane societies across America have lessened the suffering of millions of animals. For those reasons, they deserve acknowledgment and appreciation. They were included in this book's title because, unfortunately, too many refuse to recognize the real problem, which is pet breeding, and have instead looked to adoptions, and adoptions only, to solve the pet overpopulation problem.

Whether it pertains to a family pet or a Midwestern puppy mill, the urgent need to limit and regulate pet breeding has been neglected by too many humane organizations and the billion-dollar pet breeding industry has therefore gone unchallenged, and innocent dogs and cats continue to die.

What can I say about Linda Reinwand? The short explanation would be just to write "ditto." Anything I have done, she has done. For thirty-two years, Linda worked in a managerial position for Prudential Insurance Company and The Animal Birth Control Clinic would, most likely, not exist without the pristine bookkeeping and managerial skills she has provided for the past thirty-five years as the volunteer clinic administrator.

Together we formed the Humane Society of Lawton-Comanche County and, over the years, we've cried more tears than either of us want to recall due to the euthanasia of beautiful dogs and cats simply because, due to excessive pet breeding, there are too many dogs and cats in America.

We have both spent our adult lives fighting for anti-breeding laws to end, once and for all, the pet overpopulation insanity in this country.

I have depended on Linda to read either sections of this book or the entire book multiple times to search for any mistakes I may have made in that no one knows the history of the battle of the Animal Birth Control Clinic better than Linda.

She is a friend, a colleague, a fierce fighter for animals and a believer in the solutions to pet overpopulation that are espoused in this book.

I thank our past and present employees at the clinic, to include Pascall Osborne and Susan Barmettler, who have been with us for more years than I can remember, and Stephanie Chapman and Rebekah Roman, who are the newest members of our team. These employees, and their love for animals, as well as their understanding of the importance of their jobs, make the clinic the huge success that it is for all these years.

I am grateful to the tens of thousands of responsible pet owners of Southwest Oklahoma for entrusting the clinic with their pets and supporting us in difficult times, especially in the case of the most recent investigation of the local animal shelter when our name was dragged through the mud by a corrupt investigator of the Oklahoma State Board of Veterinary Medical Examiners.

AUTHOR'S NOTE

One of the most important points that anyone who reads this book must know is that it is not about revenge. It is simply the story—my story—of how I, by accident, became involved in the never-ending plight of homeless and abused animals and my shock at how so little has changed in over a century.

I have, out of necessity, mentioned names of well-known people in this community and beyond, who are an integral part of this story, some of whom are no longer living. But nothing I have written is by any means about revenge.

There will surely be those who disagree, or even be angry, with what I have written and that is their privilege. But I have told the story that I have lived—without malice or revenge. It is simply the truth.

Bless the beasts and the children; they have no voice, they have no choice.
— Anonymous

INTRODUCTION

"It is a riddle wrapped inside a mystery within an enigma"
— Churchill on Russia

THE TITLE OF this book may be a misnomer. It is, ultimately, the story of a humane movement that, like Churchill's description of Russia, is riddled with complexities, ambiguities, and misplaced priorities. It *is* an enigma.

It could, just as accurately, have been entitled *A Lost Cause* or *Hopeless* as it is the tale of a national disgrace that has spanned decades and inspired charitable giving in the untold billions, yet there is no consensus among humane societies, animal control agencies, municipalities, and certainly not veterinarians, to end it. It embodies the age-old axiom that defines insanity as doing the same things over and over again and expecting different results.

It could, *rather,* be a tale of politics, ignorance, and greed.

This story is taken from gut-wrenching personal experiences as a volunteer for over thirty-five years in the field of animal welfare. It takes to task the veterinarian community, not only for its refusal to lend its professional credibility to address the pet overpopulation and animal killing insanity in this nation, but for its intimidation and harassment of those members of the profession who *get it,* and are willing to join the effort to resolve it.

Dr. W. Marvin Mackie understands the historical culture of veterinarian resistance to low-cost spay clinics. "It's a professional embarrassment," he said in a phone conversation. Dr. Mackie has specialized in high-volume, low-cost neuter/spay clinics in California since 1976.

This book questions the mentality of a fragmented humane movement, steeped in complacency, almost devoid of innovative thinking, and so incapable of understanding *simple mathematics,* or *the law of supply and demand,* as to embrace no-kill shelters while arguing that *mandatory* neuter/spay laws are a waste of time. The no-kill proponents maintain that *voluntary* neutering and spaying is the way to address the overpopulation problem. Tell that to the puppy miller with five hundred breeding dogs in his barn and ask him when he plans to *voluntarily* make an appointment to have his "pets" neutered and spayed.

Finally, this book calls for a complete cultural overhaul of the way we think about pets and pet ownership in this country, and an unprecedented restructuring of our laws—*or lack of them*—governing unlimited pet breeding, which is, after all, the ultimate culprit.

AMERICA HAS A decades-old pet overpopulation problem. Companion animals. Dogs and cats. Animals who once ran free in the wild. Then we, human beings, domesticated them, brought them into our homes, allowed them to sleep in our beds, and made them members of our families. These wild beasts, ultimately, came to be considered *man's best friend.*

Then we abandoned them to reproduce by the millions without foresight or thought for their futures. And the best remedy that we, as a compassionate, civilized society, could come up with to deal with an overpopulation of our nation's pets has not been, simply and logically, to restrict their reproduction.

No. We deal with the problem in the most heinous, unthinkable manner possible. *We kill them.*

I WAS TAKEN aback with a question posed to me by an acquaintance I had asked early on to read the first fifty pages of this book.

"What are you trying to say, Deloris? What is the point of your book?" she asked.

She, of all people, should have understood. She had seventeen rescue dogs in her home at the time, and my first contact with her was when she had handed me a note at a city council meeting. It was 2007, and Lawton had just passed a bare knuckles, no-holds-barred, mandatory neuter/spay law. It was not unlike the hard fought law that passed back in 1992 which had never been enforced due to veterinarian opposition and politics.

The short message was hand-written on a piece of yellow note paper and simply said: "Dear Deloris, You don't know me, but you know my husband. We just wanted to say *thank you* for all your hard work involving the recent spay/neuter law. Thank you! Thank you! Thank you!"

She and her husband, a well-known former state legislator, had attended all the council meetings and used their influence with council members to get the law passed.

I thought, for sure, she understood the issues of pet breeding and pet overpopulation; and I *had* asked for her honest opinion. I should have been ready for it.

"Just in one sentence, what are you trying to say?" she pressed on. "You know, they always want you to be able to condense what you are trying to say into just one sentence."

"Oh. Uh, I don't know," I stammered. "I don't think I can put it into just one sentence. It's too complicated." I was totally flabbergasted. I made a lame attempt to explain.

"It's about dogs and cats dying, and pet breeding, and veterinarians refusing to help, and humane societies not working together, and the fantasy of the no-kill movement, and so much more."

She said my references were from too far in the past: Dr. Lloyd Faulkner's quotes taken from the 1971 issue of the *American Animal Hospital Association Bulletin* regarding spay clinics, wherein he admonished veterinarians to stop fighting the clinics and help staff them; Dr. Gordon Robinson's article from a 1990 issue of *Veterinary Economics Magazine* on "How to Keep a Humane Society Hospital out of your Community;" and other documents I had used as well.

"Well, I guess I have a lot of work to do," I conceded. "Because if you don't get the point and you think the information is outdated, then I suppose others may have the same opinion."

I hung up the phone—*devastat*ed.

Is my story old news? *Am* I hell-bent on exacting revenge on the veterinarians who had so strongly opposed us in every humanitarian effort we attempted so long ago? Was what happened to us here in a small town in Oklahoma, back in the mid-eighties, just an isolated event that never happens in the rest of the country?

I thought about this woman's criticisms. I remembered I had warned readers up front that this story *is* complicated—*that it is an enigma*. Emotions run rampant. Politics prevail. If one hasn't lived this story, then it may indeed be hard to understand. I'm not even sure I completely understand it, but from the time I first dipped my toe in the murky waters of pet overpopulation, I have known that something is wrong in this country. Something is terribly wrong. I thought again about Dr. Faulkner and his article written in 1971—*forty-nine years ago*. If you just look at the date, then you could easily think it is outdated information.

But what you have to know is that *not much has changed*. Dr. Faulkner knew that. Those were the first words out of his mouth in a phone call I made to him thirty years after that article was written. "*Not much has changed, has it?*"

Yes, due to the emphasis on the importance of neutering and spaying and the existence of mandatory neuter/spay laws throughout the nation, too many of which are not adequately enforced, and, believe it or not, exempt professional pet breeders, they have, undoubtedly made a difference in the killing statistics.

But the question is: What is an acceptable number of homeless animals and animal shelter killings? Is it the twenty million that was estimated in the seventies, or is it five million, seven million, or even the 780,000 that was a 2017 estimate. As I write in this book, I personally am convinced there is still no accurate record keeping in American shelters on a national level and no matter what website you visit, or to whom you speak, everyone has a different number for animal killings in America—because no one knows for sure. And, in my opinion, one healthy dog or cat that must be euthanized because of pet overpopulation is one too many!

BILLY, A LOCAL painter, has artfully adorned many walls for me over the years and when he is working for me, we find we have a lot to talk about.

I was surprised to learn he had, for a short time, worked for a large animal veterinarian when he was only sixteen, and he had always had an interest in veterinary medicine. I told him about the book, and he was, not surprisingly, puzzled by its title. But, unlike the woman with seventeen rescue dogs, Billy has no pets in his home, and knows little about the issue of pet overpopulation.

I gave him a quick quiz. "What if we gathered five people in a room. One of them a nurse, a plumber, a lawyer, a veterinarian, and a painter. And what if I asked which one would be most likely concerned about the welfare of animals. Which would you choose?"

Billy said the answer was a no-brainer. "The veterinarian. Of course."

If you are reading this book, you probably have at least some interest in the world of animals. You most likely own a dog or a cat or, like many of us, multiples of both. America is a nation of pet lovers. Celebrities lend their names to large organizations, such as the ASPCA or the Humane Society of the United States, for fund-raising purposes.

Howard Stern, the Sirius radio shock jock, and his wife, Beth, to their credit, foster cats for the North Shore Animal League, and Stern offers them up for adoption on his radio show.

A few years ago, I came across a new cable station called DOG TV. From a couple of weeks of free programming, I was able to glean that the primary purpose of DOG TV is to transmit into our homes scenes of grassy meadows, and clear blue streams, purely for the viewing pleasure of our dogs while we are away from home.

I considered DOG TV, but I couldn't get even one of the seven dogs who live in my home to commit to a viewing preference. Did they like DOG TV? Or did they prefer Anderson Cooper on CNN? Maybe they just wanted to keep up with the Kardashians. How could I tell? They couldn't be bothered to lift up their heads from the dog beds and couches on which they were sleeping.

Maybe I hadn't given DOG TV a real chance. I had only scanned over it once or twice. And I *am*, after all, writing about it. I needed to do my research; and it was only five bucks a month. I picked up my phone and called Direct TV. As quick as I could say *ridiculous*, there on my screen was a program entitled "Afternoon Stimulation." A click of the info button informed me these were "programs to increase mental and physical stimulation for dogs when home alone."

On another day, as I was flipping through the channels, I came upon a show called *Too Cute* on Animal Planet. This programming was simply dogs and cats, of all shapes and sizes, posing or frolicking for the cameras, with sounds of music wafting softly through the air.

I wouldn't even attempt to deny that those visions of soft, fluffy, wide-eyed canines and felines were indeed *too cute,* just as the show's title implied. But I'm not into fluff. I'm hard core. I've seen the dark side of America's fascination with its pets; and it's not cute.

Some might consider hard core the aforementioned ASPCA television ads, where homeless dogs and cats gaze sadly into the TV camera as Willie Nelson croons, "You Are So Beautiful," or Sarah McLachlan sings, "In The Arms Of An Angel." These ads *are* certain to bring tears to your eyes, and send you straight for your checkbook.

But I am Pistol Pete with the remote when these ads hit my TV screen. I see enough abandoned animals in my everyday life, and I don't want to see any more unless it's for a purpose better than fund raising. I know that billions have been donated—*over decades*—on the backs of these helpless animals, and nothing really changes.

I want ads such as these to *inform* Americans what *they* can do to end the plight of these helpless animals.

Use this valuable nationwide TV opportunity to tell viewers to be sure their own pets are neutered and spayed. Convince them never to perpetuate the overpopulation of dogs and cats by *buying* from a *pet shop* or a *breeder.*

Plead with them to help end pet overpopulation by adopting from their local animal shelter when—*and only when*—they decide they can responsibly take care of a pet.

Finally, and most importantly, tell America it is crucial that we have, throughout this nation, laws that restrict and regulate pet breeding, and that are strongly enforced, in order to—*once and for all*—end this American disgrace.

Then I'll make a donation. *Maybe.* But probably not. Because I know that several of these huge organizations, while asking you for your money to care for an *overabundance* of pets, are, at the same time, astonishingly, opposed to anti-breeding laws. Besides, I need to keep my donations right here in my *own* community, at the grassroots level, where overworked volunteers, without the benefits of plush offices and corporate-type salaries, struggle daily on shoestring budgets, and a never-ending stream of needy animals in search of a good home.

I'VE SAID THE words *pet overpopulation* so many times in my life, it sounds commonplace. Almost boring. Probably not words of such significance as to awaken the conscience of a nation.

Would a more trendy label get the attention of a complacent society? I doubt it. But I am lacking for a better choice of words. Animal overproduction? Excessive pet breeding? American insanity? A solvable problem? It's all of those things—and more.

Pet overpopulation is a big enough problem to shut down the mass transit system of the nation's largest city a few years ago in order to spare the lives of two stray baby kittens.

But there are communities all over this nation who *wouldn't* have stopped the train. There is no animal control in huge sections of the United States. Many farmers and rural animal control officers shoot stray dogs on sight, and drown baby kittens and puppies in gunnysacks.

Killing. Euthanasia. Call it what you will. *Humane or otherwise,* it's the number one cause of death in dogs and cats in America, far surpassing the toll taken by common diseases seen by veterinarians in their daily practices.

Mandatory neuter/spay laws. Do they work? Could they stop the killing? What does mandatory even mean when it comes to neutering and spaying of dogs and cats?

When I began to research the hundreds of these laws in municipalities across the country, I was shocked to learn just how many loopholes are in many of these laws. The animals that are exempt *alone* would create a massive overpopulation problem—even if every single other animal that falls under the law were neutered and spayed.

Some of the exemptions include animals that compete in shows or sporting competitions, guide dogs, animals used by police agencies, and those **belonging to professional breeders.**

Did I read that right? Animals belonging to professional breeders are exempt? The natural enemies of any type of breeding or "litter" laws, as I prefer to call them, **are exempt?**

What happens in states like Oklahoma is that legislators see the puppy mill dog breeders the same way they see farmers. They view the dogs like cattle and the good ole boys are just "makin' a livin.'" Perhaps, in these cases, even if the government has to pay the puppy millers *not to breed* (choke) until they could make arrangements to make a living in another manner, the same way farmers have been paid *not* to plant certain crops, then so be it.

If the government paying breeders not to breed would end this national insanity of killing beautiful innocent pets for no other reason than just being born, then let's get out the checkbook. It's a start.

How tough would it be to get a national moratorium on pet breeding until supply equals demand? Damn tough! It would be the battle of the ages. And it would require animal advocates to be on the same side. And therein lies the problem.

It is what it is, and whatever we choose to call it, pet overpopulation is animal cruelty at its worst. It's animal cruelty at our own back door, and *veterinarians, humane societies and others* have come to accept the killing as just the way we do things in America.

CHAPTER 1

"The worst type of crying wasn't the kind everyone could see–the wailing on street corners, the tearing at clothes. No, the worst kind happened when your soul wept and no matter what you did, there was no way to comfort it. A section withered and became a scar on the part of your soul that survived." — Katie McGarry, *Pushing the Limits*

HISTORICALLY, ACTIVISM HAS irked those in positions of power in all levels of government, as well as special interest groups, and there is a price to pay for being outspoken for a cause.

First, you lose your anonymity. That was not something I ever relished. I just understood that it goes with the territory.

Being passionate and vocal cuts two ways. You gain the respect of those who agree with you and the wrath of those you are offending. To some, you are a hero who could walk on water while others wish you would drown. But there is always a price to pay.

"THAT WILL BE fifty dollars," said the young woman behind the desk in the city clerk's office.

I arrived at Lawton City Hall early that Thursday morning in March 2015. I was anxious to purchase my copy of the just-released report of the two-month investigation of wrongdoing at the Lawton Animal Shelter.

The City of Lawton had requested the services of the Oklahoma State Board of Veterinary Medical Examiners to conduct the investigation, oddly enough, with the urging of Councilman Keith Jackson, much to the chagrin of many of us who knew that the investigator, as well as the OSBVME, had a serious conflict of interest in multiple areas.

I wrote a personal check and handed it to the clerk behind the desk. "Have you sold many copies of this," I casually inquired.

"No. You are only the second one," she replied.

As I waited for her to prepare my receipt, I gently turned over the cover of the report to the index and the first few pages, and as I did so, a wave of nausea came over me.

"I don't believe this," I said, speaking more to myself than anyone else. "I do not believe this."

I saw my name everywhere. And associated with my name, I saw words like conspiracy and defendant. I also saw the names of others, good citizens of Lawton, who had spoken out against the cruelty and mismanagement that was entrenched in the daily operations of that facility.

The woman behind the desk had nothing to say to me. She seemed to have no curiosity or interest in my distress. Perhaps she knew.

She handed me my receipt and I hurried down the long corridor of the recently remodeled building to the elevator that would take me one floor down and to my car.

Once in the sanctuary of my perpetually cluttered Hyundai Genesis, an emotional dam broke, releasing a river of tears that could no longer be contained.

I called Linda.

"Oh my God, Linda," I wailed in full-blown sobbing mode. "It's worse than we ever thought it would be."

Still on the phone to Linda, I started my car and headed to Jackson's Laundromat.

AS I LOOK back, the tell-tale signs were everywhere that the tax-supported shelter was not what citizens thought or wanted to believe it was. For my part, the pain and perplexities associated with the cause of animal welfare only served to compound the gut-wrenching, soul-penetrating pain and sorrow I was experiencing at that time as my beloved cancer-stricken, terminally ill daughter, Dana, was dying.

IN AUGUST 2016, in the wee hours of the morning, with a broken ankle propped on a pillow and surrounded by five dogs (two of the seven had died of old age) I was soul searching in a small bedroom at the home of Jamie, my youngest daughter.

I found myself reflecting on my life, still agonizing over my daughter's death in October 2015, while at the same time learning to live my life in what Hospice describes as a changed reality, a process of which there is perhaps no end. I was also seeking desperately, along with other named defendants and conspirators who had been so maligned by the City of Lawton and the Oklahoma State Board of Veterinary Medical Examiners, to understand what had happened here in Lawton in March of that same year. And why?

"I am bereaved, wronged, homeless, and footless," I mused to myself with a mixture of self-pity and sarcasm. Actually, I wasn't footless. That, I assume, would imply that one has no feet. I had fallen and broken my ankle and, for all purposes, I might as well have been footless in that I wasn't going much of anywhere for at least twelve weeks. And I was only somewhat homeless.

On June 12, 2016, the creek that surrounds my country home and had been the symbol of peace and beauty that I had loved for decades, betrayed me and with the fiercest force of nature came rushing through my home taking with it a lifetime of memories.

My oldest son, Monty, and I, along with a few friends and neighbors, entered the house on that Sunday evening.

"I feel like the house has died," I told Monty later that night as we drove away from the devastation. Dana is gone and now the house is gone."

Actually, I was lucky compared to others in Lawton. My home received only around nine inches of water while other homeowners in Lawton barely got out with their lives with water up to their rooftops. A dam on a lake at the nearby military base had broken and that, coupled with a huge amount of rainfall, had produced what some were describing as a five-hundred-year flood. The house can and is being fixed. And I was able to recover some of my cherished possessions. I was able to save perhaps as much as I lost.

As I was self-assessing and pondering the events of the past year, I recalled the strange words of Dr. Reynolds when I had learned about an article in the *Wall Street Journal* regarding the calcium chloride neutering of dogs at the Lawton Animal Shelter.

Dr. Reynolds performed surgery for more than twenty years at the Animal Birth Control Clinic, a high-volume, low-cost neuter/spay clinic founded in 1985, much to the chagrin of Lawton veterinarians and the Oklahoma State Board of Veterinary Medical Examiners. Although he no longer performs surgeries, he is on hand on off-surgery days to handle vaccinations.

Clinic employees Susan Barmettler and Pascall Osborne had shown me the internet article dated November 28, 2014. The piece was entitled "Too many Dogs: A Simple Solution." Written by Melinda Beck, it discussed the pros and cons of using the experimental solution for neutering male dogs, especially on Indian reservations and third world countries.

The last paragraph is what had prompted clinic employees to bring the article to my attention. Beck wrote that a few U. S. Vets and shelters "are quietly starting to use calcium chloride. Rose Wilson, who supervises an animal shelter in Lawton, Okla., has been using the drug since last spring, with the blessing of city officials. She says that she wouldn't go back to surgeries. 'We haven't seen any problems with it,' she says. 'It's simple, it's inexpensive, and it's painless. This is the best thing that's happened in the spay/neuter world in a long, long time.'"

"Quietly" was the key word in the article. Few, if any, Lawton citizens knew of the use of this experimental chemical at our tax-supported shelter. Once it was brought to light, citizens did complain as there were indeed plenty of complications and dogs were dying painful deaths. The city manager put a halt to it as a result of the complaints.

"Why wouldn't Rose have said something to me about this?" I asked Susan and Pascall. "I don't understand this. Why would she not have said something to me?"

Rose had called me a few years before to ask my opinion on selling the corpses of cats to a company for research. I had agreed that the animals were already dead and I could see no reason not to do it. In my opinion, it was a way to increase the budget, which I erroneously believed could and would be used for the welfare of the live animals at the shelter.

As late as 2014, when the article was dated, we had discussed pet overpopulation on multiple occasions and both agreed that the no-kill movement could not and would not solve the problem. It had only been a few months earlier that she had called me about the Fort Sill military base situation wherein city and state neuter/spay laws were not being enforced at that facility. I believe Rose believed, as a city employee, she could not address the situation so I had stepped in and placed phone calls to people on the military post and at the Pentagon.

I simply couldn't understand it. I knew nothing about calcium chloride neutering. Nothing. Because of that I would not have immediately objected to it. Rose knew about my lifelong commitment to reduce pet overpopulation and why wouldn't I be interested in something that was cheaper and simpler if it was indeed safe? In fact, she had heard me complain that the veterinarian community had done little to advance safe and innovative methods of animal birth control.

I should make it clear that Rose was not, in any way, obligated to share any aspect of her job with me. I merely felt we had some sort of relationship, even if it is hard to describe. And, after all, her job and the animal shelter were tax supported.

There were no clients in the clinic at the time, and Dr. Reynolds was sitting at a desk in the surgery room where he overheard the conversation. He is a tall, rather reserved man with a quiet, slow manner of speaking. He walked into the prep room and came over to where I was standing next to the prep table. As he towered over me, in almost a whisper, he shocked me with his words.

"They didn't tell you about this because they don't like you," he said. "They don't like you, they have never liked you, and even though they may be nice to your face, they will never like you."

I was shocked at his explicitness. I wasn't sure whether or not he had just hurt my feelings.

"You mean they don't like me or they don't like this clinic?" I asked.

"They don't see any difference," he answered.

The question as to who "they" were didn't come up. But we both knew. The veterinarians would never forgive me for the low-cost neuter/spay clinic and a Federal Trade Commission ruling years before in 1989. And we both knew that Dr. Wayne Haney, who was performing the experimental calcium chloride neuters, was one of the earliest and most vocal opponents of the Animal Birth Control Clinic thirty years earlier.

And Rose herself most likely resented the fact that too many people reported to us what they saw or experienced at the animal shelter. We would learn later from two whistle blower shelter employees that Rose did indeed immensely dislike those of us at the Animal Birth Control Clinic.

We were just too damn meddlesome!

YES, HISTORY HAS proved over and over again that there is a price to pay for being vocal for a cause.

And this was not my first payment.

CHAPTER 2

"Well-behaved women seldom make history." — Laurel Thatcher Ulrich

"GET OUT OF the car, lady."

"Why, what did I do?"

"Get out of the car!" the angry police officer demanded a second time.

I stepped out of my husband's blue Nissan pickup onto the gravel parking lot of a brick company that ran parallel to Gore Boulevard, on which I had been driving. I was blinded by the overhead flashing lights of four patrol units that were surrounding me. An all-points bulletin had been transmitted over police radio to stop my vehicle. The scene could just as easily have resembled a police response to a tip on a serial killer.

"Get out your license," the officer ordered.

I reached for my handbag, fumbled for my wallet, and produced my Oklahoma driver's license.

"Run this," the officer said, as he handed my license to one of the four officers.

The officer, who I later learned was Lt. William Mathis, walked over to where I was standing and came up very close to me. His index and middle fingers were tightly clenched together.

"Let me tell you something, lady," he growled, shaking his fingers up and down in my face. "I don't care who you are, or who you think you are, you're not going to call down there and talk to me like that," referring to a phone call I had made to the police station only moments before.

I was thinking to myself about the condescending behavior of this policeman; and I was comfortable in the knowledge that I had done nothing to break the law. Perhaps, in retrospect, I should have toned down my response. However, as I have read over mounds of court documents as research for writing this book, I feel certain I would behave no differently today. I had called the police station for information, provided my name, and, initially, behaved politely.

I looked squarely back at Lt. Mathis. "Well, let me tell you something. I don't care who you are, or who you think you are, I'm a taxpayer and a citizen, and you're not going to talk to me like this."

The officer said that there are eight city councilmen and a mayor and a city manager here, and if I didn't like the way they do things at the police station, I should call them, but I wasn't going to call him and complain "like that."

"I ought to take you to jail right now," he threatened.

I remember thinking this guy doesn't even know the number of council members in the City of Lawton, which were ten at that time; and he was talking about taking me to jail. For what?

"Well, why don't you just do that," I argued, "if I've done something to warrant you taking me to jail, but I'd like for you to show me where it's written, in the state statutes or the city code, that I can't call the police station, and question the actions of an officer, or complain about one."

"I don't have to show you anything," Mathis retorted.

Lt. Mathis and I didn't know each other. We knew about each other. He perceived me to be a woman of privilege, with time on my hands, running around town, getting into other people's business—i.e. the business of the police as it related to the animal shelter. A woman would later testify, in court, that Mathis had told her I was a well-known, long-time trouble maker in Lawton.

I knew him to be a rogue cop who had shot in the back and killed, a young, shirtless, barefoot, unarmed, African American boy who was fleeing for his life. But I had never seen him before that Saturday night, and I didn't know who he was at the time.

I also knew that two animal control officers, who were affiliated with the police department, had been fired only two weeks earlier as a result of a horrific act of animal cruelty. I had not kept silent in the matter and Lt. Mathis set out on that balmy July night in 1992, surrounded by his uniformed minions, amid their pulsating, cherry red lights, to see to it that this well-known, long-time trouble maker in Lawton got her just dues.

Even back then, I had already learned many times over that standing up for what's right often has repercussions. But little did I know just how serious those repercussions could be until twenty-three years later when a twisted and bizarre turn of events involving an animal shelter once again steeped in horrific acts of animal cruelty, and an investigation of that shelter with its entangled web of lies and cover-ups, left me and other Lawton citizens stunned, with our First Amendment rights violated, and wondering just what the City of Lawton, Oklahoma, had to hide.

Actually, for Linda and I, it was just another case of déjà vu.

CHAPTER 3

"'So tell me, since it makes no factual difference to you and you can't prove the question either way, which story do you prefer? Which is the better story, the story with animals or the story without animals?' Mr. Okamoto: 'That's an interesting question.' Mr. Chiba: 'The story with animals.' Mr. Okamoto: 'Yes. The story with animals is the better story.' Pi Patel: 'Thank you. And so it goes with God.'" — Yann Martel, Canadian Author, *Life of Pi*

IT WAS THE mid-seventies, and my late husband, Dan, and I were about two miles outside the city limits of Lawton, a military town with a population of just under 100,000, when I spotted a beautiful piece of land on a corner adjacent to a heavily tree-lined creek.

Without thinking, I blurted out, "Wouldn't this be a beautiful place to have a home and raise our kids?"

We were not on a mission to buy land. We simply had a rare couple of hours to ourselves, and had taken a drive out into the Oklahoma countryside. It was a beautiful spring afternoon. The Oklahoma wind, made famous by Rodgers and Hammerstein's Broadway play, was noticeably absent. The road was flanked on either side with a glorious array of dandelions, yarrow, Indian paintbrush, and black-eyed Susans. There was a certain feel in the air that day, and the longer I looked at that beautiful spot, and the more I thought about it, the better I liked the idea of life in the country.

I knew nothing about gardening, but I was conjuring up images of a vegetable garden, an organic one, of course, with the compost heap and the whole nine yards. I was visualizing myself lying in a swaying hammock, tied between two of those huge old trees, with trickles of sunshine beaming through the branches. I was a dreamer all right. When does a mother of four ever find herself lying in a swaying hammock?

I actually was surprising myself. I had grown up in the country for the first thirteen years of my life, and, if I recall correctly, swore I never wanted to go back to it.

LIFE IN THE late thirties and early forties hadn't been particularly great. There had been the depression, which I hadn't fully comprehended, except to know that we were poor. But so was everyone else. Then there was the war. Most kids back then understood at least something about the war because we had fathers or brothers who were away; or a mother or sister who was a Rosie the Riveter, a woman who worked in a defense plant building war paraphernalia.

The depression and the war aside, a bedfast and terminally ill father from the time I was eight until his death when I was thirteen, brought about hardships early on. We lived on a farm with cows, and our source of income was selling bottled milk in our small rural community.

Every morning my mother and I would awaken at the brink of dawn and set about hand milking what I recall to be about twenty cows, but was probably only eight or ten. The milk went into glass bottles, and before I went to school, we drove our old jalopy around town and I jumped in and out, delivering our freshly bottled milk all over the tiny rural community of Elgin, Oklahoma.

When my father died, my mother and I moved to what, in my young mind, was a city. Actually, it was a town of about two thousand people. I swore then I had left the country life for good.

But something was coming over me on the drive that day, and the country life was once again beckoning. What is that old adage? You can take the girl out of the country, but you can't take the country out of the girl.

I spotted a farmhouse about a quarter of a mile down the road. "Pull up to that house," I said to my husband. "I'll just get out of the car and ask if there is any land out here for sale. What can happen to me for just asking?"

The door of the old stone house slowly opened, and a tall, stately looking man, who appeared to be in his early seventies, peered out the door. "What do you need," he said in a cordial enough voice, probably assuming we were having car trouble.

I pointed to the piece of land by the creek. "I just told my husband the spot on that corner down there would be such a wonderful place to build a house," I said, somewhat sheepishly, considering I had awakened him and his wife from their afternoon nap. "Do you have any land out here for sale?"

To my surprise, he invited me in. Grinning and proud of myself, I motioned to Dan to get out of the car and come with me. The farmer introduced himself. His name was Don Harvey and he and his wife, Sava, were polite and surprisingly sophisticated. They both had been in Lawton for most of their lives.

They told us how their family had owned the local movie theaters back in their day, and that their only living relative was a son who was in California and had no interest whatsoever in coming back to live in Oklahoma.

We continued to talk over glasses of iced tea, and, finally, we got back to the subject of the land. They admitted that, due to aging, they had indeed been thinking about selling some land.

To our utmost surprise, they agreed to sell us the land that was our chosen spot. It was twelve acres of a former alfalfa hay field, which lay in a pie shape on the northwest corner of their farm.

In the years that followed, we became friends and neighbors with the Harveys. Five years after our purchase of the twelve acres, when they felt they had no other choice than to move into a high rise apartment for senior citizens, they offered us the remainder of the hundred-and-sixty-acre farm.

A little over a year later, after that spontaneous Saturday afternoon drive, Dan and I, and our four children, moved into the new home in the country, which we believed would be our place of solace, our shelter from the storm, our refuge from the world. And even with the creek's bouts of flooding over its banks, on occasions of heavy rain, this home has been all of those things—with one exception.

Although my husband was a businessman operating a successful Nissan dealership, and our children, with their usual teenage idiosyncrasies, were not overly problematic, our lives would prove to be anything but carefree in our new country home.

As I look back, I wonder if our lives, my life in particular, would have taken a different direction if we had chosen to live within the city limits; or, at least, somewhere other than the Oklahoma countryside—perhaps in the tiny ski resort town of Alta, Utah.

CHAPTER 4

"There are a hundred million dogs and cats in America. We cuddle them, talk to them, make them part of the family. Every year we buy them $5 billion worth of food, not to mention collars, bowls, flea spray, vaccinations and little pink sweaters. We love our pets. Except of course when we have to move, or get tired of walking them, or sick of paying the vet bills. Then we abandon them. By the millions. We tell ourselves they'll find a new home, but the truth is when we drop them off at the animal shelter, we drop them off to die." — John Dorschner, "See Spot Die" *The Miami Herald*

"THERE ARE TWO dogs in the intersection outside your house," the voice said on the other end of the line. It was a neighbor who lived about a mile to the north. I didn't know her name. She had driven right past the two dogs, but was concerned enough to at least make a phone call.

I went outside to have a look and, indeed, there were two dogs no older than six months wandering around the intersection. Their owner obviously thought they would stand a better chance on a gravel rural road than at the city animal shelter. And this time, at least, these two little dogs did beat the odds that were stacked against them.

I called to each of them and one, who later became Trixie, a small black and white terrier, readily came to me. The other one, a long-haired, brindle-colored mix with a turned-up tail, was terrified and headed for the ditch.

I went into the house and came back with food. The two dogs were half starved and as Trixie started to chow down, Ubu, as the brindle was later named, couldn't resist. He left the ditch and headed for the food. After about an hour of coaxing, I was finally able to get both of them into the house. Ubu and Trixie lived out their lives as part of our family, as would many others who would come after them.

FROM THE TIME we had first moved to the country, we were inundated with countless numbers of stray dogs and cats who wandered up to our doorstep. Others had to be fed on the side of the road until we could catch them. Oftentimes, we were forced to resort to setting humane traps, which could take hours or days.

I spent almost all of my time, and a tremendous amount of money, attempting to find homes for these abandoned pets.

My knowledge of the overall problem of pet overpopulation was as limited back then as is that of most average Americans today.

In my ignorance, we bought a Collie puppy from a breeder and then allowed Lassie to have her own litter of puppies, encouraged by the advice of a veterinarian who recommended dogs have at least one litter for the sake of health. Some veterinarians actually believed that in those days. I placed Lassie's puppies into homes wherein I would never place them today.

In a matter of months, a litter of eleven puppies were dropped off at our front gate. I needed to find homes. One of my children's classmates wanted a puppy. Did he have his parent's permission? Who knew? I didn't bother to find out. I didn't know about cat traps back then and an employee of my husband's car dealership wanted a kitten from a litter of a mama cat we couldn't catch. Would this be a good home for the kitten? I had no clue.

These were homes. Never mind that I had not screened them nor did I know if they would be permanent. I had neglected to demand they be spayed or neutered when they became old enough so they wouldn't reproduce and perpetuate the problem I thought I had just solved. I didn't bother to check and make sure that these helpless animals would not once again be tossed out onto some country road. These were homes. And I was out of space in my home.

Although it is no consolation to me whatsoever, I was not alone in my ignorance. For decades, the "free to good home" message has appeared in newspaper classifieds, on bulletin boards of laundromats, feed stores, veterinarian offices, and anywhere such messages can be posted. An accidental litter of kittens; a litter of puppies born just for fun for the children's education and entertainment; a nine-year-old Golden Retriever who's become incontinent; a move to an apartment that doesn't take pets; or a military family assigned to a new post.

Due to the easy availability of an overabundance of dogs and cats in this country, too many Americans change pets as often as they change hairdos, wardrobes, or automobiles. Based on my own experience, I would be willing to bet my bottom dollar that in nine out of ten cases, there is no screening of potential adopters that result from these advertisements. God only knows where and under what conditions the free to good home pets, those unwanted, disposable castoffs, spend—and end—their lives.

I make it a point not to go to PetSmart, and other stores, on adoption days. I know many pets end up in good homes from those events, but I also know that many of the candidates for adoption have been in foster homes for long periods of time. And then, as quick as a six-year-old can say, "Mommy, can I have that doggie or that kitty?" they leave the security of that foster home and become victims of an impulse, unscreened adoption—and often end up right back in a shelter again.

So many times I have wondered what happened to those pets that I personally had handed out like candy bars to just anyone. On a couple of occasions, I found out; and it was heartbreaking.

"Do you still have that kitten we gave you?" I quizzed a radio advertising sales rep one day at the car dealership.

The pretty blond looked puzzled. "You know," she said whimsically, "I don't know what ever happened to that cat."

I was devastated to learn that the employee who had adopted another kitten had no clue as to its whereabouts. He had literally tossed it out the front door when it had a bout of diarrhea.

"I put it outside and never saw it again," he told me. He couldn't have been more nonchalant.

AS THE ANIMALS kept coming, homes for them kept drying up. I couldn't accept the option of humane euthanasia back then some thirty-five years ago. We adopted many of the animals ourselves, so many that our lives were upside down. We continued to hound our friends to take others. The expense was tremendous. I was replacing carpet every couple of years. We eventually replaced every square inch of a five bedroom house with wood or tile floors that could be washed. The area rugs that hadn't been chewed up or peed into oblivion had long been put away, and years later given to our son and his wife. I like to think that I am, at least, of average intelligence, and it didn't take me long to realize that the answer to too many dogs and cats is not in finding homes that just don't exist. We don't need an economist, or a mathematician, to explain to us that when supply far exceeds demand, things get out of whack; and, in the case of dogs and cats, the ending is not a happy one.

Unregulated pet breeding can be likened to an open water faucet that has been flowing for over a century, and, rather than turning off the faucet to deal with an unending stream of water, the best solution anyone has devised is to convince friends and neighbors to take the water into their homes—one bucketful at a time.

This is the case with the huge "no kill" movement in this country, which can never become a reality until we first address the unending flow of puppies and kittens into the American marketplace.

Pet overpopulation takes a toll on human lives as well. Too often, animal rescuers, who cannot—or will not—come to terms with the unfortunate necessity of euthanasia, wind up in the poor house, overwhelmed with more pets than they can feed or care for properly. The next thing you know, they're labeled animal "hoarders" or "collectors," and someone is having to rescue animals from the rescuers—usually with television cameras rolling.

CHAPTER 5

"We live in a world which is full of misery and ignorance, and the plain duty of each and all of us is to try to make the little corner he can influence somewhat less miserable and somewhat less ignorant than it was before he entered." —Thomas H. Huxley, English Biologist

"I GAVE THESE people a donation today," Dan said as he handed me a crudely made flier that had been given to him by a couple of women who had solicited a donation at the car dealership that day.

"Hey, this is great," I said, as I looked over the brochure. I was overjoyed at the thought of a new animal organization in town. At that time, there was no humane society in Lawton, or, for that matter, for miles around. The local animal shelter was a stepchild of the police department, and horror stories of animal abuse ran rampant.

The group was called VAPS. It stood for Volunteers for Animal Protection Society. I could tell my husband and I were thinking the same thing. We'll make nice donations, they'll take the strays who come to us, and life will be normal again. Problem solved!

I wanted to help this new group be successful in any way I could. I found my way onto their board of directors. On that board also were two Lawton veterinarians.

I did what I could to help this struggling organization survive. I made donations, published a newsletter for them, and hosted a fund-raiser at our home, at which several thousand dollars were raised. During this time, I had taken a couple of stray dogs to them to be adopted.

By this time, I had grown at least somewhat in my knowledge of the pet overpopulation problem. I certainly knew that there were more animals than homes. I knew that somehow animals in my community had to be "fixed." And I had become painfully aware of my own mistakes in adopting to just anyone who would carry the pet away.

I attended board meetings and was disappointed to learn that animals were being placed into homes just willy-nilly. Record keeping was sporadic and, in some cases, the names of adopters were unknown. I had already been there and done that, and I wanted no part of repeating my same mistakes.

I also was questioning the sincerity of the veterinarians on the board. Sometimes I wondered if perhaps they were there to control rather than contribute. But why was I so suspicious? They were veterinarians. Their first concern would be for the animals, wouldn't it?

Today, as I look back on those times, I still find it strange that I had that sixth sense, or mistrust, so early on, in what would, only a few months later, become an all-out war.

My suspicions were justified in the months to come. One of the doctors would indeed become a thorn in our side, at every turn, for years to come. And while the other one joined the opposition early on, he moved on, and is today the doctor to my own family pets.

The VAPS organization was laden with problems. I learned one of the founders had accepted the care of a dog that belonged to a military family, and was in quarantine awaiting release to join its owners in Germany. They had given VAPS money to be used for their pet's air fare to Germany, however, a VAPS volunteer had used the money for her own personal use. To save face, we, the board members, voted to contribute money to get the dog to its owner.

By now, my interest in this organization was not just waning; it was ended. This was not a problem-solving group.

So much for VAPS.

The VAPS organization stayed in Lawton a number of years, and there were good people in their organization who tried to do their best for animals. They were adamantly against euthanasia, and their sole function was animal adoptions as is the local humane society here in Lawton today.

As for me, I was back to square one.

CHAPTER 6

"It is common sense to take a method and try it. If it fails, admit it frankly and try another. But above all, try something." — Franklin D. Roosevelt

"LINDA, THIS IS Deloris Delluomo," I said into the phone. "I'm having a meeting at my house Tuesday evening at seven. I want to talk about forming some kind of animal organization. I don't mean a humane society, as such. Not necessarily one that adopts out animals either. We just need something that addresses the problem of all these strays we have out here."

Linda Reinwand is my neighbor who lives just over a mile from my house. She worked for thirty-two years in a managerial position for Prudential Insurance Company. Our children had played together, and gone to the same school. We were, however, at that time, more acquaintances than friends. She and her husband had also been dealing with strays for years, and she, too, was ready to see if we could find a solution.

She has not left my side since, and, over the years, together, we've climbed over barbed wire fences—one that Linda learned the hard way was electrified—to rescue dogs; scaled trees to rescue cats; crawled under buildings to rescue mommas with litters of puppies and kittens; gone on cruelty calls in the middle of the night; set traps for strays we couldn't catch; and been arrested while doing so. Okay. I'm the only one that's been arrested—not Linda. With the help of our husbands, we've gone to small towns in Oklahoma we'd never heard of and picked up stock trailer loads of dogs that had been abandoned at empty farmhouses. On one bizarre occasion, in the middle of winter, we rescued three dogs who were tied to trees in a desolate wooded field in two feet of snow.

We've cried more tears than we want to recall, as we held perfectly beautiful dogs and cats in our arms, while the needle of death went into their veins, simply because, due to excessive pet breeding, there are too many dogs and cats in America; and not enough homes.

Linda would become secretary-treasurer of the new organization that would come out of that meeting, a position she still holds today. As a part of those duties, she would become the volunteer administrator of The Animal Birth Control Clinic, a high-volume, low-cost neuter/spay clinic, which arose from the ashes of our attempts to involve local veterinarians in a community effort.

I SET OUT cookies, cold drinks, and coffee for about nine people who had gathered in my living room on that Tuesday evening in November, 1984. Even though the Oklahoma fall weather was still mild, Dan had built a cozy fire for us in the stone fireplace. We settled in to discuss the problem at hand.

I began the conversation. "I've talked to veterinarians in this town who tell me they are neutering or spaying only one or two animals a week, or even less."

I knew a few of the veterinarians in our community. In fact, they actually liked me at the time. What was not to like? I was a client rescuing animals who needed veterinary care—lots and lots of dollars worth of veterinary care.

Little did we know that, within months, I would become the Dragon Lady, worthy of mention, if not the topic of discussion, at a local Comanche County Veterinary Medical Association meeting. "What are we going to do about Deloris Delluomo?" According to word on the street, that was the question posed by Dr. Dan Woesner at that meeting.

Our group discussed the fact that our community and our state are low on the socio-economic scale. Oklahoma is ranked as one of the poorest states in the nation, and we concluded that most likely the reason pets weren't getting neutered and spayed was because their owners couldn't afford it. Our later research proved that to be the case across the nation. It remains true today.

A valid argument could be made that those who can't afford to have a pet neutered or spayed simply should not have a pet in the first place; but that scenario would only be true in a perfect world—not the one in which we live today.

One by one, my guests began to speak about how a world overpopulated with homeless dogs and cats was affecting their lives.

"My friends hate to hear me calling anymore," Sherry Tilley said. "I've used them all up for homes for strays. My house is full, and my husband is frustrated."

Sherry lived in a fantasy world. Like most of us at that time, she wouldn't hear of euthanizing a healthy animal just because it didn't have a home. She truly believed she could care for every animal that came her way, in spite of limited financial means and a small manufactured home at one of the nearby lakes.

"I think there are a lot of people here who will help us," Sue Neal said enthusiastically. Sue never met a person who intimidated her. She has always been outspoken, bold, and energetic, with her heart in the right place. We immediately placed her in charge of fund raising.

I hear from Sue once or twice a year. She is in a small community near Canton, Texas, which is home to one of the most infamous flea markets in the nation. It is a veritable breeder's pet-trading extravaganza. When the flea market days are over, scores of unsold pets are abandoned on the county roads, and Sue is drowning in the middle of all that.

Occasionally, she will drive to Lawton to bring two or three new dogs to the clinic to be neutered or spayed.

"I'll probably still be crawling under fences to rescue dogs when I'm eighty," Sue posted on social media recently. No joke. Things need to change soon, as Sue is in her seventies now.

"Gandhi said you can gage a civilization by the way it treats its animals, or something like that," Marne Botkin said in her high-pitched girlish voice.

Marne was a free thinker, a Bohemian-type soul with a deep love for animals. She, too, had too many strays, and not enough funds, and wouldn't hear of euthanasia. We made her vice president of public education.

Maureen Oehler, now Maureen Durant, was Dana's best friend since childhood. Maureen isn't an animal lover. Her calling has always been to teach. She is a wonderful high school and college educator, extremely civic-minded, and she offered to help.

Maureen's stay with us was, however, short-lived, as she married the love of her life, Brian, and moved to West Point, New York, with her military husband. Upon Brian's retirement, they have relocated back to Lawton, and I have sought Maureen's expertise as a testing ground for this book. In other words, I forced her to read it.

Kay Jenkins was also a school teacher, and she and her husband, Gene, and their children, were our closest neighbors at that time. They were also having their share of problems with stray dogs and cats, and she was more than anxious to join our group.

A husband and wife couple, who shall remain nameless as it serves no purpose to name them, also seemed eager to attend that first meeting. At that time, we obviously knew very little about their beliefs, but they must have convinced us they were on board with everyone else's philosophies, because we made one of them vice-president of neuter/spay programs, and the other vice-president of animal shelter/city involvement.

Those appointments would later on prove to be a problem. As we came to learn, weeks into our program, this couple believed in neutering and spaying of other people's pets, as long as they were not purebred, and as long as they didn't belong to them. We also discovered they were actually purebred cat breeders, an activity that was completely antithetical to what we were trying to accomplish.

By the end of the evening, we had all overwhelmingly come to the same conclusion: We could not in a lifetime find homes for all the abandoned animals with which we were all dealing. This organization would have to be dedicated to problem-solving, which meant reducing the number of homeless and unwanted dogs and cats. And that could only be accomplished by a massive, no-holds-barred, community neuter and spay project.

We could do that, couldn't we?

What, or who, was there to stop us?

ALL SORTS OF names for the organization were bantered about. We finally settled on The Lawton United Volunteers for Animal Birth Control. Lacking in brevity, but explicit.

We were incorporated under Oklahoma laws on November 29, 1984, with the purpose and objectives being legislation, education, and sterilization, an adaption of the LES program as outlined several years earlier by the Humane Society of the United States.

The IRS granted us a 501c3 status several months later.

We ordered every piece of literature available on the subject of neutering and spaying pets to reduce an unwanted pet population.

Arming ourselves with information on "How to Establish Spay and Neuter Programs and Clinics," we set out to establish the cooperating veterinarian program. Local veterinarians would reduce their neuter/spay fees, and our organization would, in turn, conduct outreach and public awareness campaigns, resulting in high volume surgeries. The high volume of surgeries would compensate veterinarians for their reduced fees.

We sincerely had a big tent philosophy in those early days. Subsequent meetings were held with attempts to bring in all the veterinarians, who were also asked to serve as honorary members on our board, but with no votes.

Thank Heaven, we were smarter than that.

CHAPTER 7

"The legitimate cost of current technology . . . is undoubtedly beyond
the means of a segment of our society which may have genuine
needs for pet ownership . . . Is the waiting list for low-cost ovario-
hysterectomies limited to indigent widows and children with pets? Not
on your life, doctor." — Dr. Lloyd Faulkner, "Spay Clinics," *American
Animal Hospital Association Bulletin*, Autumn 1971

KAY JENKINS AND I sat waiting in the small office of Dr. Don Beavers,
president of the Comanche County Veterinary Medical Association. We were
surrounded by framed degrees, pictures of family, and other mementos. We
giggled at the doctor's hunting trophies.

"I guess when he's not healing animals, he's out shooting them," we chortled.

This was, at the time, my personal veterinarian. He listened to our concerns
and was courteous. We left there, however, without any commitment whatsoever
of local veterinarian involvement.

"I thought we might have had him there at one point," Kay said as we were
getting into the car to leave the clinic. "I thought he might come on board and
agree to help us, but I don't think so now."

"Yeah," I agreed, "I didn't see a lot of hope there."

Having received no verbal commitment of involvement, our next step would
be to outline a formal written proposal to present to each local veterinarian. The
Proposal for Veterinarians in Community Neuter/Spay Programs was sent to the
fifteen local vets on January 31, 1985.

Our research had revealed that veterinarians participating in high-volume,
low-cost neuter and spay programs, or neuter/spay clinics—wherever we could
find them, as they were sparse in those days—were performing sterilization
procedures for an average overall fee of thirty dollars.

The gist of the proposal was that participating veterinarians agree to
"standardize their neuter/spay fees at thirty dollars for all candidates, male or
female, dog or cat, making no distinctions as to clients to whom lowered fees
would be available."

In return for reduced fees, our organization would "solicit neuter/spay
candidates through aggressive multi-media advertising, door-to-door canvassing,

and direct telephone survey, and would subsidize payment, when necessary, as long as the participating veterinarian charges the reduced fee of thirty dollars for all neuter/spay surgeries."

We asked the veterinarians to return their yes or no responses by February 12, 1985.

FEBRUARY 12 ARRIVED, and we had heard nothing. We waited another week or so. Still nothing. In the meantime, we had been promoting our new organization, and people were starting to send us donations to be used in neuter/spay projects.

After approximately another week, I called Dr. Beavers. "I'm wondering why I haven't heard something back from anyone. Does this mean you guys don't want to help us?"

"No one wants to spay or neuter anything for thirty dollars," was his response. "If your group could subsidize our prices, that would be a different situation."

"By subsidize, what do you mean?" I queried. "Are you not willing to lower your costs at all?"

This doctor was a slow-talking, fairly quiet-spoken individual—a likeable guy. He explained the position of the veterinarians very calmly.

He went on to propose that they would continue to charge the same. Our organization could subsidize those prices with fund-raisers and private donations.

"So, in other words, you wouldn't be contributing anything?" I asked. "You would have increased volume, an opportunity for new clients and other procedures, but you wouldn't be contributing anything? To a community effort?"

I stopped for a moment. "You know, Don, we have little old ladies sending us five dollars out of their Social Security checks because they believe in what we're trying to do. I just can't, in good conscience, use their money that way."

There was silence for a moment, and then I spoke again. "So, I guess I know where we stand." The moment was awkward. But I never knew when to quit.

"I don't think any of you want to see a low-cost spay clinic here in Lawton, do you?"

"No, I don't think any of us want that," Dr. Beavers said.

Before we ended the conversation, I made this doctor of veterinary medicine a promise. "We're going to have affordable neuters and spays in this community one way or the other," I said politely—but firmly.

And if a spay clinic is what it takes, then a spay clinic is what it takes.

CHAPTER 8

"We must concede, I think, that at least we have no suitable technological alternative, and spay clinics are a positive measure toward the solution of an immense problem, albeit unacceptable to the profession of veterinary medicine." — Dr. Lloyd Faulkner, "Spay Clinics," *American Animal Hospital Association Bulletin*, Autumn 1971

REFUSAL OF THE veterinarians to work with us came as no surprise. They had already begun to get nervous when VAPS formed, and especially so during my stint with that organization, inasmuch as my chosen role with them was to promote neutering and spaying.

It was no secret they had historically found ways to prevent Ft. Sill military veterinarians from performing elective surgery, including neuters and spays.

At one point, I became worried that local veterinarians would refuse to treat my own pets. My vet, however, continued to treat my animals, and Dr. Joe Kelsey, who was closer to the Elgin area than Lawton, was always kind and helpful. At one point, he said to me, "I don't know what their problem is," referring to the opposition we were experiencing from Lawton veterinarians.

By now, word of this new, aggressive organization was buzzing all over town. The words neuter and spay were becoming as familiar as Pepsi and Coke.

We set up booths at local events, delivered fliers, ran public service announcements on local radio and TV stations, and had another large charity picnic and auction. Not a day went by that we were not delivering the neuter and spay message.

A couple of redneck wise guys in a local bar described me as "the bitch who wants to get everything neutered." They actually weren't far from wrong. My cohorts and I were becoming fanatical neuter and spay advocates; and the harder the veterinarians pushed back, the stronger we pushed forward.

"LINDA," I SAID, "we're going to have to open our own neuter/spay clinic. The vets are never going to work with us."

I had called her at her job at Prudential that day in February 1985, after Kay Jenkins and I had been to see Dr. Beavers.

"How in the hell are we going to do that, Deloris?" Linda asked in a panicked voice.

"Well," I said, "it's gonna mean a whole lot of garage sales; and Dan has agreed to co-sign a bank note with us."

It's not clear how local veterinarians, at that time, were able to exert so much influence on the military veterinarians at Ft. Sill.

What they were about to do to us was another story. It is the story on which this book is based.

OKLAHOMA VETERINARIANS HAD, for years, governed their own under the Oklahoma Veterinary Practice Act with a set of Rules of Professional Conduct that prohibited a veterinarian working for anyone other than another veterinarian.

"It shall be dishonest for a licensed veterinarian to accept employment from a non-licensed person, company, firm, or corporation for the sale of his professional services to the public . . . Every licensed veterinarian shall be governed and controlled by the Rules of Professional Conduct adopted by the Board . . ."

Thus, a veterinarian, under the rules of conduct, could not work directly for humane organizations in a clinic, or on any projects no matter how badly they were needed.

It never occurred to us that a veterinarian would not be allowed to work in our clinic. If we built it, they would come. That was our logical assumption. We were oblivious to the Rules of Professional Conduct of the Oklahoma State Board of Veterinary Medical Examiners in Oklahoma City. But these rules would become their strongest ammunition against us—their veritable ace in the hole.

One fact was indisputable. Not one of the members of our group could perform a neuter or a spay if our lives depended on it. Ironically enough, we were going to have to have a veterinarian. What a perplexing state of affairs in which we were about to find ourselves.

We were, however, undaunted in our passion and zeal. "Who could actually stop us from opening a spay clinic?" we asked ourselves. This is America! Remember? Capitalism! Free enterprise! Walmart!

At this point, it was a matter of educating ourselves on just how one goes about setting up a surgical veterinary facility. What the heck was an autoclave? What instruments go into a spay pack? What is a spay pack? What constitutes a bank of stainless steel cages? Shoreline. Suburban Surgical. Smith Klein Beecham. Pfizer. Who sells what?

We called for the help of the late Toni DeStephano, executive director of the Wichita County Humane Society, which was fifty-five miles away in Wichita Falls, Texas.

"I want this to succeed," Toni had told me. "You call me anytime. I'll do what I can to help." Their clinic had been up and running in Wichita Falls for several years. From Wichita Falls to Waco, our Texas neighbors were good to us in those days.

Dr. Roger Harlan, of the Dog, Cat, and Bird Clinic in Oklahoma City, was sympathetic and helpful to our predicament. He, too, had suffered from veterinarian harassment, as he, himself, was performing low-cost neuters and spays at the time. Throughout the years, I have not forgotten his willingness to talk to me at any time, and advise us on surgical equipment, instruments, medicines, and suppliers.

In spite of how hard it was going to be to pay for it, we always bought the best clinic equipment available. We opted for the digital tabletop read-out scale, whereas we could have used a much cheaper and less sophisticated scale. These days we have the walk-on digital scale, which is back-saving for employees handling the big dogs.

We chose the top-of-the-line Shoreline hydraulic, V-top surgery table, but could have done well on a much less expensive model. We literally wore that old table out a few years ago, and a California foundation, who stipulated the name of the foundation nor the celebrity who funded it, could not be used in any publication, provided us with a grant for a brand new V-top, hydraulic surgery table, but this time a heated one. They also provided the walk-on scale and multiple other replacements of old surgical equipment.

Over the years, it has been imperative that we dispel any rumblings about "getting what you pay for," or "cutting corners" at our clinic.

It was bad enough that clinic personnel at one of our bitterest opponents in town—it just happened to be the doctor who was on the board of VAPS—has had a habit of telling people our clinic performs surgeries without anesthesia.

Really? Just how would you manage that on a seventy-five pound unfriendly pit bull?

Customer after customer, however, has come into our clinic throughout the years, telling us that tale, so it must be true—not the part about the anesthetic, but the rumor. Even to this day.

A few years ago, I happened to be in the clinic in the front reception area, and I noticed an older dignified-looking man, dressed neatly in jeans and a short-sleeved, button-down shirt. He had no animals with him, and he said nothing.

He just seemed to be taking in what was happening around him. A couple of other customers were getting vaccinations for their dogs.

"Sir, have you been helped?" I asked.

"I'm just here to see the setup and ask a few questions."

"Maybe I could answer something for you," I proposed.

He was quiet spoken, perhaps even timid at first. "I have a friend who lives in the country, out by Anadarko, and he has a lot of strays dumped out by his house. I try to help him with the expenses of getting them fixed. I just paid a hundred and fifty dollars for a spay to a clinic on the other side of town. I can't afford that, with so many animals to fix, and I had heard about this place, but I'm . . . well, I'm just here to check things out."

I decided to help him out. "Have you heard things like maybe the animals are not anaesthetized for surgery?"

He seemed relieved that issue was out in the open. "Yes. I did hear that. But as I am looking around, I see this is a first class place, and I would imagine that's not true."

I told him I knew where he had gotten that information. It was the same place where his last dog had been spayed. It was the clinic across town.

"I'd like to use this clinic," he said almost apologetically. "But I just want to be sure it's on the up and up."

I invited him to take a tour of the clinic. I walked him back into the surgery room, then the prep room, then showed him the wall of shiny stainless steel cages, all lined with soft bedding and waiting for the next day's patients.

"They're all wrapped up in those blankets as they are waking up from the anesthesia," I said, bringing home the point.

The two of us must have talked for about an hour. He was a very intelligent man. We talked about politics, the environment. He was extremely savvy with regard to the overpopulation problem and steps that must be taken to end it.

He booked an appointment for his neighbor's latest stray that same day.

This man and his friend, who exhibit so much kindness to animals that have been abandoned, warm the heart. In spite of the odds against them, they are doing what they can.

Contrast their attitudes with the farmer who drove up to the clinic with a dog in the back of his pickup truck.

"Someone dumped this dog out on me and if you don't take it, I'm gonna shoot it," he threatened. We took him seriously. We took the dog.

Early on, we countered the untruths about the clinic with ads that read: "Our low-cost fee includes two nights board, and all the tender loving care your pet can stand from people who love animals."

WE HELD FUND-RAISERS of every kind imaginable to finance our project. Our frequent garage sales, which were held at the car dealership, became almost famous. They were huge, thanks to so many donations from Lawton citizens. Automobiles on the showroom floor were replaced with used furniture, clothing, odd sets of dishes, and dozens of used sets of sheets and bedding donated by a local hotel. Our garage sales were events not to be missed.

At the fund-raisers, we would take the name of each person and ask questions such as "Do you own a pet?" "Is it neutered or spayed?" "If not, then why not?" "Would you do it if the costs were lower?" In almost every case, the answer to the last question was a resounding "yes."

CHAPTER 9

"We are tardy in enlisting the capabilities of the profession in support of the cause of the humanists . . . We can scream that spay clinics are . . . an encroachment upon professional domain and private enterprise. I think that would not solve any part of the pet population problem and would be to the detriment of the profession . . . I would encourage the profession to take every possible means to cooperate in attacking the problem at all levels . . . In the meantime, it may be wise to help in staffing the spay clinics until more suitable procedures are available."
— Dr. Lloyd Faulkner, "Spay Clinics," *American Animal Hospital Association Bulletin*, Autumn, 1971

OUR ADVERTISEMENTS PROMISED the clinic would be open May 1, 1985, just three months after I promised my veterinarian a spay clinic in Lawton. When that date rolled around, however, we weren't quite ready. One critically important aspect of our program was missing: a veterinarian.

Yes. We had no veterinarian. And we had more than a hundred surgeries tentatively booked. We didn't receive a single call, or resume, from ads placed in the campus newspaper at Oklahoma State University School of Veterinary Medicine at graduation time.

I did hear about one local woman who was graduating with a DVM degree from OSU. It seemed worth my time to, at least, give her a call.

I introduced myself and congratulated her on her degree from OSU.

It quickly became obvious I had lost her at hello. "Thank you," came the cool reply.

"You may or may not have heard that we are opening a neuter/spay clinic here in Lawton?"

"Yes, I have heard that," she said.

I was getting nowhere.

"I was wondering if perhaps you might be interested in working with us. Do you like to do surgeries?"

"Oh, I could never do that to the veterinarians in Lawton," came her quick response. "I've known some of them for years, and I just couldn't do that to them."

I quickly and politely ended the conversation, hung up the phone, and sat stunned. What the hell?

We actually got calls from a couple of out-of-town vets who were willing to work with us. But, in many instances, they were too far away in distance to be comfortable with regard to possible postoperative complications.

In spite, however, of days when our future seemed hopeless, our work seemed to have a guardian angel hovering nearby all along. In fact, unbeknown to us, what was to come our way a few years down the road was nothing short of a miraculous divine intervention.

IT WAS AROUND the middle of May, 1985. Dan and I were at a restaurant in town and ran into Dale Coody, a local farmer.

"I hear ya'll are looking for a veterinarian," he said in his natural Oklahoma drawl. He told us about Dr. Jeff Tidwell, who lived in a community about twenty minutes away, and who might be interested in working at our clinic.

I wasted no time. I contacted Dr. Tidwell that same afternoon, and he did indeed agree to perform surgeries at the Animal Birth Control Clinic. He was a young, topnotch veterinarian and surgeon.

Things were looking up.

We opened for business on May 23, 1985, just three months after we'd failed to engage local veterinarians in our cause—with a hundred surgeries on the appointment book.

On that first surgery day, Dr. Tidwell revealed that he preferred to sit down while performing so many surgeries.

I jumped in my car, zoomed over to the Nissan dealership, and ran into the parts department.

"I need this," I said, grabbing a barstool from the counter.

"I'll explain later. Don't have time now," I yelled, running out the door dragging the stool, leaving behind a puzzled-looking parts manager.

I rushed the stool over to the clinic and placed it right next to the surgery table. Just perfect. In a low-cost neuter/spay clinic, embroiled in controversy, it was the least I could do for a young veterinarian who had just walked himself smack dab out on a limb.

I'M NOT SURE how long it took for Dr. Tidwell to receive his first letter from the Oklahoma State Board of Veterinary Medical Examiners, wherein he was advised that his license would be in jeopardy if he continued to work at the Animal Birth Control Clinic. But it didn't take long.

He was able to stave off the wolves at the board for a short period of time, but no veterinarian who has spent all that money, and all those years in school, wants to lose his or her license, no matter how frivolous the complaint against them.

The letters he received from the Board, and subsequent ones to subsequent veterinarians, read almost the same: "The Oklahoma State Board of Veterinary Medical Examiners has reviewed the complaint against you by the Comanche County Veterinary Medical Association concerning your employment by the Lawton United Volunteers for Animal Birth Control for the sale of your professional services to the public.

" . . . You are hereby ordered to terminate those aspects of your practice which violate the provisions of this Act and to forward to the Board a letter stating the date by which you will be in compliance."

Thank you and goodbye, Dr. Tidwell.

IT'S INTERESTING TO note that at almost the exact moment in time, veterinarians in Pennsylvania were having their own problems with a troublesome humane society, who obviously also wanted to see a reduction in dead animals in their community.

In the Law Notes section of the Fall 1985 edition of the Humane Society News, published, at the time, by the Humane Society of the United States, an article was entitled: "Veterinarians Sue to Close Spay-Neuter Clinic."

The article stated that four individual veterinarians, along with the Northeastern Pennsylvania Veterinary Medical Association, had sued to stop the Humane Society of Lackawanna County, Pennsylvania, from owning and operating a veterinary clinic. The suit charged the humane society with "unlicensed practice of veterinary medicine; violation of state corporation law; intent to monopolize the rendering of veterinary services in the local market through deliberate price cutting and saturating the market with advertising; and unfair competition with commercial veterinary hospitals by treating animals below reasonable cost."

The complaint alleged, according to the article, that HSLC, because of its operation of the clinic, had no valid claim to its exemption from federal, state, and local taxes and was, therefore, soliciting tax deductible donations improperly and illegally.

The article stated that veterinarians have asked the court to "enjoin HSLC from any further operation of the clinic and to order HSLC, whose services were limited to spaying and neutering operations, to return all fees earned from the clinic."

I did my best to learn what had become of that litigation. Numerous calls to the Humane Society of Lackawanna, Pennsylvania, proved unfruitful. The same was true with the Humane Society of the United States, where it was all but impossible to speak to a live person.

As it pertains to this book, what is important to know is that the Humane Society of Lackawanna County, Pennsylvania, was sued by veterinarians in their community simply for getting dogs and cats neutered and spayed—a practice that saves millions of dogs and cats from death.

That type of veterinarian harassment continues today throughout the country.

As this is written, neuter/spay clinics in Alabama are fighting for their right to exist.

CHAPTER 10

"This nation is spending hundreds of millions of dollars annually in a losing battle. Relatively nothing is expended on research to find reasonable alternatives. . . ." — Dr. Lloyd Faulkner, "Spay Clinics," *American Animal Hospital Association Bulletin*, Autumn 1971

THE SECOND VETERINARIAN on the scene was Dr. Larry Chambers. I can't recall exactly how or when he became involved, but I am certain he contacted us. We would not have contacted him inasmuch as he was, and is, a local veterinarian with his own practice; and we knew where local veterinarians stood on the issue of this clinic. I have never been sure why he came to work for us. Perhaps it had to do with our pay scale, which was not half bad due to a high volume of surgeries.

I do know that his first letter from the Oklahoma State Board of Veterinary Medical Examiners was dated June 13, 1986. It read the same as Dr. Tidwell's letter: "You are hereby ordered to terminate those aspects of your practice which violate the provisions of this Act and to forward to the Board a letter stating the date by which you will be in compliance."

Dr. Chambers attempts to assuage the board's demands obviously failed.

It was Wednesday, July 2, 1986, in the late afternoon when Dan phoned me from the car dealership.

"There's an article in the Constitution that says the clinic is closed," he said.

"*What?*"

The local newspaper was always delivered to the dealership, not our home. In those days, there were two editions each day. One was the evening Lawton Constitution and the other was the Lawton Morning Press.

"I'll be right there," I said.

I rushed into my husband's office and grabbed a copy of the newspaper. Sure enough. There it was in bold headlines: "Animal clinic temporarily closed."

The first paragraph of the article stated: "An order from the state board governing veterinarians has temporarily shut down a low-cost animal sterilization clinic here, but the founder of the clinic has vowed she will keep it in operation."

That was interesting. I had not had a call about this from the newspaper nor anyone else. And one thing was certain. The Animal Birth Control Clinic was not closed.

In fact, the cages were full of animals that had come in that day waiting to be neutered and spayed the next morning.

"Dr. Larry Chambers, the veterinarian contracting with the clinic operated by the Lawton United Volunteers for Animal Birth Control, said Wednesday he will end his contract with the clinic on Friday," the article stated.

Might have been nice to have given us a heads up, Doc.

The now familiar litany of the Board's Rules of Professional Conduct was printed verbatim. The article went on to quote Dr. Michael Benham, then secretary of the board of examiners: "Enforcement of the law is not an attempt to suppress competition between veterinarians and such low-cost clinics but is aimed at protecting the integrity of veterinarians and veterinary medicine.

"The board of examiners is not in the business of creating monopolies for vets," explained Dr. Benham.

Oh yeah?

The article outlined the policies of the clinic explaining that the "charges for spaying or neutering an average-sized animal was $30.00, about half the charge of local veterinarians for the surgery. The clinic also has a policy that no animal will be turned away, regardless of the ability of the pet owner to pay for the surgery." That part was at least accurate.

WHY AT THIS point was I not feeling defeated? The newspaper had pronounced us closed. Local veterinarians and the OSBVME were never going to leave us alone. Where would we find a steady stream of new veterinarians as current ones were intimidated and forced to leave?

Somehow, I was not defeated. I was mad. My first call was to the newspaper. I don't remember my exact words to them, but I'm certain they were anything but polite.

In the meantime, the animals were in the cages in the clinic awaiting surgery on Thursday morning. That's when I received the call from a panicked clinic employee.

"Dr. Chambers is not going to show up!"

Now, I am a high-strung, anxious, sometimes annoying, specimen of the Homo sapiens species given to bouts of panic in a high tense situation. How I was able to refrain from running out of my house, with my hands in the air and my hair on fire, I cannot say.

But, strangely enough, that did not happen.

THAT SAME DAY, Thursday, July 3, 1986, the evening Constitution printed
a retraction of the information from the previous day's paper. This headline read:
"Founder says clinic to stay open."

"A story and headline in the Wednesday issue of *The Lawton Constitution*
indicated that an order from the state board of veterinarians had temporarily
shut down the clinic. The statement was in error."

You bet it was in error. By the time that newspaper hit the streets, all of
those twenty dogs and cats, who sat waiting, were already neutered and spayed—
without Dr. Larry Chambers. We understood the doctor's need to protect his
license. It would have just been nice if he had talked to us first.

Again, the newspaper outlined the fees, and even the clinic hours. Actually,
thirty years later, when I'm not so mad, I think those articles provided excellent
free advertisement for the clinic.

Maybe kind of like divine intervention.

But this was just a small insignificant divine intervention. The big one was
yet to come.

CHAPTER 11

"It is an insult to my integrity to assume that I, or any other veterinarian who is in good standing with the OVMA or the AVMA could not maintain professional ethics, no matter whether the pay check was coming from a private individual, another veterinarian, or a client." — Dr. Becky Brewer-Walker in a letter to the Oklahoma State Board of Veterinary Medical Examiners, August 15, 1986

"DR. BREWER, I'M with the Animal Birth Control Clinic in Lawton, and we are in a bit of a predicament here," I said into the phone.

From somewhere, I had obtained the name of a veterinarian from Chickasha, a small town located about forty minutes away from Lawton.

Her name was Dr. Becky Brewer-Walker. We called her Dr. Brewer or Dr. Becky.

"I don't believe we've ever met, but I understand you do relief work around the state, and we could really use some help here today," I said, hoping she would detect the desperation in my voice.

Could she come today? Could she come now? "Please. Anything you can do," I pleaded. The short story is that she came. She came that very day. All those animals, waiting in their cages, were safely neutered and spayed.

Dr. Brewer came on subsequent surgery days, in the interim, when we were without a permanent veterinarian. In spite of the local newspaper reporting we were closed, and Dr. Chambers walking out on twenty scheduled surgeries, we didn't miss a beat. We never have.

Dr. Brewer worked for us until August 8, 1986. Whether or not she received a letter from the Board is unclear. She, however, wrote her own rather sassy, albeit respectful, letter to them dated August 15, 1986. She explained to the Board that she performed euthanasia for the City of Chickasha animal shelter. She defended the work of the clinic as a means to address the unfortunate killing of excess pets. She was adamant that she would keep the Animal Birth Control Clinic on her relief list.

IN SPITE OF veterinarian protests and newspaper gaffes, we had support from citizens and other media outlets. On March 7, 1986, I wrote a letter to Ms. Pat Pitts of KSWO TV thanking her for a PSA her station was running on behalf of our organization.

"The spot is extremely well done and obviously very beneficial to our cause as we have received numerous calls from pet owners inquiring about, and booking, neuters and spays," I wrote.

"For those of us . . . who cannot thank you for themselves, we wish to express our deepest appreciation to you and the staff of Channel 7 for your support of animal welfare causes."

It's important to note here that, actually, throughout the years, the Lawton Constitution has been somewhat supportive to the animal cause in a variety of ways. It's been a mixed bag. On the one hand, they have printed most of our letters to the editor—often after being pressured to do so; allowed us to write op-ed pieces—once to counter an ugly personal attack on me by, of all people, their sports editor, who I had never met. They have carried our press releases; and covered stories about animal issues in the city. Columnist Paul McClung wrote a great article about pet overpopulation and the new Lawton United Volunteers for Animal Birth Control early on. But, on the other hand, they have sided with the veterinarians in every single battle that has been waged—and there have been many!

ENTER DR. ZBIGNIEW Richard Zdunek. We received Dr. Zdunek's resume in early August. We signed an agreement wherein he would lease the clinic equipment, which was more a technicality than anything else. Anything to placate an ever-threatening veterinary medical board.

There was, however, no appeasing the Comanche County Veterinary Medical Association or the Oklahoma State Board of Veterinary Medical Examiners.

Dr. Zdunek endured the wrath of the CCVMA and the OSBVME, and was able to dodge their bullets for approximately eighteen months.

And then, alas, when he had endured all he could endure, he took his leave to quieter, less stressful employment environments, away from the City of Lawton.

IN LATE 1987, Kenneth L. Reynolds, D.V.M., M.P.H. presented us with an impressive resume. It was impressive, not only in veterinary medicine, but also in human disease, ranging from studies at the Centers for Disease Control in Atlanta, Georgia, to a three-year stint as Chief of Veterinary Medicine at the Eisenhower Army Medical Center in Augusta, Georgia. He had published papers on everything from Pediatric Infectious Disease to Emergency Medicine, and Cancer Research in humans.

Dr. Reynolds had filled in for Dr. Zdunek, who was on vacation for a couple of weeks in December 1987. He started full time in April 1988.

The Animal Birth Control Clinic and Dr. Reynolds were a match made in heaven. Our surgery room was akin to his man cave. He was at a point in his career where he was happiest spending most of his time in surgery, rather than meeting pet owners and diagnosing disease. Our surgery numbers were growing by leaps and bounds, and his pristine surgical skills were just what we needed.

Bending over a surgery table for twenty years, however, took its toll on Dr. Reynolds' neck. He gave up the surgeries in 2008, but remains with us to the present in order to administer vaccinations on off-surgery days.

Wait a minute. Did I just say Dr. Reynolds performed surgeries at the Animal Birth Control Clinic for twenty years? Did he not get letters from the Board? Was he not harassed in the same manner as all the other veterinarians?

Yes. Yes. And, hell yes! Relentlessly!

So just how did he manage to get around those pesky OSBVME Rules of Professional Conduct that stated he couldn't work for a non-licensed person or organization—for twenty years?

Did I mention I believe in divine intervention?

CHAPTER 12

"First they ignore you, then they laugh at you, then they fight you, then you win." — Mahatma Gandhi

IT WAS SPRING, 1988, when the first call came from the Federal Trade Commission. I was standing at the counter in my kitchen when the phone rang.

"May I speak to Deloris Delluomo," the voice said on the other end of the line.

"Yes, speaking."

Back then, we didn't have cell phone appendages as part of our bodies. Except for what we referred to as "car phones" that required plugging into the automobile's cigarette lighter, we used land lines.

"This is Kristin Malmberg with the Dallas Regional Office of the Federal Trade Commission." The Federal Trade Commission? Holy shit! What now? I needed to sit down. I pulled out a chair from the nearby kitchen table.

She asked if I was president of the organization that operates the Animal Birth Control Clinic. "Uh . . . yesss."

Questions were racing through my mind. Can the Feds actually come after you for starting a low-cost spay clinic?

Ms. Malmberg said she wanted to ask me some questions. Her tone was not intimidating. She was professional and courteous. That was somewhat calming.

"Ok," I said. Whatever it was I had done, I settled in for my grilling.

It was my understanding that the FTC had been performing a routine investigation of the files of professionals in Oklahoma who govern themselves under the Oklahoma Practice Act. Upon examining the files of the OSBVME in Oklahoma City, they found a large file pertaining to the Animal Birth Control Clinic in Lawton. I can't say whether or not the ABC Clinic was the commission's sole reason for instigating the investigation. I do know that we were a big part of it, and I can only report that Ms. Malmberg told me they were investigating Oklahoma veterinarians.

"Oh, really?" I said, breathing a sigh of relief. Thank you, God. Obviously I wasn't the one in trouble after all.

Ms. Malmberg was interested to know about our attempts to get the veterinarians to work with us on the neuter/spay project.

Her primary question was whether they had answered our letter individually or as a group.

I told her everything I knew—how we had sent out the proposal letter, and got no responses, and how we had been told that no one wants to spay a dog for thirty dollars.

We talked for a while, she thanked me for the information; and that was the end of that.

In a few weeks, another call came from Ms. Malmberg. Again, the same line of questioning. Did the veterinarians respond to our proposal for help individually or as a group?

There was definitely a pattern to her questions. I finally rallied enough fortitude to ask her why that was important. She informed me they were investigating the veterinarians for possible "horizontal collusion."

"Horizontal what?"

She explained that horizontal collusion means price fixing.

Oh! Interesting.

Ms. Malmberg requested a copy of our proposal to the local veterinarians, and other written correspondence between the OSBVME and our clinic veterinarians. In each and every case, our veterinarians were essentially ordered to cease and desist their employment with the Animal Birth Control Clinic.

On one occasion, Ms. Malmberg came to Lawton accompanied by another investigator. Dan and I took the two women out to dinner at Martin's Restaurant, which, at the time, was Lawton's finest and most frequented steak house. Again, the primary topic of discussion at the dinner table was the ongoing harassment our veterinarians were experiencing from the OSBVME in Oklahoma City and the CCVMA in Lawton.

When my husband asked the waiter for the check, Ms. Malmberg hastily rejected his offer to buy dinner. She explained that it would be the same as them accepting a gift from us.

"Okay!" I was thinking to myself. "This just keeps on getting better."

It was my understanding that the two investigators also spoke to several Lawton veterinarians before their return trip to Dallas. I don't believe they ever called me again. I would, however, have an occasion to speak to Ms. Malmberg one more time, a year or so later.

But wait. I am jumping ahead of myself in this story. Long before the Federal Trade Commission would ever hear of the Animal Birth Control Clinic, or the Comanche County Veterinary Medical Association, a mass of dirty deeds and verbal garbage would wash under the proverbial bridge in Lawton, Oklahoma.

For a battle, on yet another front, was about to be waged with Lawton veterinarians. But this time, they would not be able to rely on their Rules of Professional Conduct—or help from the Oklahoma State Board of Veterinary Medical Examiners in Oklahoma City.

On the subject of honesty and integrity on the part of FTC investigators, we would see something very different in the behavior of an OSBVME investigator hired by the City of Lawton twenty-seven years later to examine its malfunctioning and corrupt tax-supported animal shelter.

CHAPTER 13

"Both sides have valid points philosophically and economically. The issue is complex and emotional. The crux of the problem to humane groups is killing animals; the crux to veterinarians is unfair tax-exempt competition." — Dr. Gordon W. Robinson, VMD, "How to Keep a Humane Society Hospital out of your Community," *Veterinary Economics Magazine*, 1990

I'M NOT THE most organized human being on the planet. That's why the clinic has Linda as administrator. She is the organizer-in-chief. But I do somehow manage to hang onto things that may be important some day in the future.

In lieu of neatly filed documents, I have plastic tubs brimming full of yellowed and fragile newspaper clippings; and correspondence to veterinarians, politicians, city officials, and at least a dozen celebrities to whom I've begged, futilely, for help.

Perhaps my most bizarre effort to capture a celebrity's attention regarding pet overpopulation was a letter I wrote to *Hustler Magazine* publisher Larry Flynt on January 11, 1997. I had caught a portion of a TV autobiography of Mr. Flynt's life, and learned of a cat he had taken home as a small boy only to have his father tell him to get rid of the cat.

Seizing on any scrap of hope this might be an animal person, I wrote to Mr. Flynt.

The letter began with the following words, bold and italicized: "Let me just spit it out up front: Would you consider using your influence to tell America that sex in human beings is great, but in America's pets it amounts to death? What an enigma if the King of Porn who has hyped sex in humans would condemn sex in dogs and cats."

Okay. So it was a crazy idea. And, alas, I never heard from Mr. Flynt, nor any of the other celebrities to whom I had written, in the hopes of bringing the national insanity of pet overpopulation to a public discussion.

In my plastic tubs, there are also USDA inspection reports on Oklahoma puppy mills, obtained under the Freedom of Information Act, copies of grant requests, and Federal Trade Commission rulings.

Anything remotely associated with the pet overpopulation problem, or animal issues in general, has, over the years, gone into those tubs.

I came across a cover story in the June 1990 issue of *Veterinary Economics Magazine* entitled "How to Keep a Humane Society Hospital Out of Your Community."

It was written by Dr. Gordon W. Robinson, then vice-president of the ASPCA in New York City and director of the Bergh Memorial Animal Hospital of the ASPCA. The magazine noted he was immediate past president of the Veterinary Medical Association of New York City, and an area director of the American Animal Hospital Association. Impressive credentials.

Dr. Robinson attempts to explain the complexities of the historical clash between humane societies and veterinarians. He admits, obviously from his own experiences with humane organizations, that humane society workers often spend most of their time killing the animals to which they have dedicated their lives.

He concedes that "humane societies need the cooperation of veterinarians to get out of the killing business. The societies don't look at it as getting into the surgery business; they look at it as getting out of the killing business."

That's it! In a nutshell. Dr. Robinson gets it!

Dr. Robinson explains the veterinarians' position: "Historically, this is where humane societies and veterinarians have come into conflict. The humane society approaches the veterinarian for cheap, discount spays. Dr. Jones is horrified and insulted by 'cheap' and 'discount' . . . This is not Kmart. I'm a professional, and professionals don't have blue light specials."

In the 1990 writing, however, Dr. Robinson admonished his colleagues to cooperate with animal welfare advocates. "Since surgery is currently the only way to do pet birth control, that means cooperate with a low-cost spay/neuter program, or they will build their own spay/neuter clinic."

"It's that simple," Dr. Robinson advised. "Cooperate or compete."

But the truth of the matter is that spay clinics, which the fictional Dr. Jones, and others, so vehemently despise, should never have become a necessity. It's folly to believe that any humane group would have chosen to enter that arena, if given a choice. It is a huge undertaking to establish a veterinary surgical facility, and even a more arduous task to operate it on a daily basis—especially as volunteers.

The veterinary community, in general, however, has failed to get it, and has refused to cooperate; and animals have continued to die—by the millions.

In the absence, i.e. disinterest, of the veterinary community to scientifically research safe and painless alternative sterilization procedures, or cooperate with humane societies in pursuing restrictive breeding laws, neutering and spaying is all we've ever had.

And that, my dear Lucinda, is how spay clinics are born.

CHAPTER 14

"The rumors you have heard about spay clinics are a good deal more than what you have perceived. The rumblings which have reached you are shock waves originating in California and, I suspect, other distant places. The profession would err grossly by mistaking these events for something which, I believe, they are not . . . Spay clinics and the problems which have led to their conception are real." — Dr. Lloyd Faulkner, "Spay Clinics," *American Animal Hospital Association Bulletin*, Autumn 1971

ALTHOUGH THE ANIMAL Birth Control Clinic in Lawton was one of the early clinics in the United States, spay clinics were not a completely novel idea at the time. In 1895, the American SPCA was drowning dogs in the Hudson River, a practice later replaced by gassing, which, sadly, is still practiced in some shelters today. According to internet statistics, the number of homeless animals killed by the ASPCA was over 100,000 in 1908, and "averaged more than 250,000 per year from 1966 through 1968, when Lloyd Tait, DVM, started the first discount dog and cat sterilization program."

However, California has historically led the nation in innovative and new age thinking, and that held true in the area of low-cost spay clinics. In 1971, the City of Los Angeles, under the guidance of Robert Rush, Director of the Los Angeles Animal Regulation Department, opened the first public neuter/spay clinic in the United States.

I had an occasion to visit with Mr. Rush on a trip to California with my husband for a new car showing in Los Angeles. While Dan attended meetings pertaining to automobiles, I met with Mr. Rush regarding neuter/spay facilities. He graciously invited me to accompany him to the opening dedication of the third neuter/spay clinic in the area.

I was privileged to be in the company of one of the earliest pioneers in the low-cost neuter/spay movement. I collected every piece of available literature pertaining to the clinics, along with copies of the City of Los Angeles' laws pertaining to animals.

I recently checked online only to discover that Mr. Rush had retired in 1992. My heart sank to read that he had been embroiled in controversy toward the end of his tenure with the City of Los Angeles. The city's six shelters at that time were reported to be in dilapidated condition, according to the 1992 article in the *Los Angeles Times,* due to "lack of funds."

A lack of funds should never be the case when it is associated with tax-supported animal shelters. Cities and counties have it within their power to enact stiff licensing, and neuter/spay laws, in the form of breeding permits and fines, that would offset the cost of municipal and county animal shelter operations—and save the lives of millions of animals. But, unfortunately, very few fight for these laws as there is no consensus among humane groups; and, the American Veterinary Medical Association, according to their website, oppose neuter/spay laws.

The article quoted Mr. Rush as saying he "couldn't take it any longer," with regard to his work in animal regulation, stating that he was suffering from a bad heart condition.

The "I can't take it any longer" syndrome is common among animal advocates and animal shelter workers, weary of the revolving door of animal abandonment and euthanasia.

Mr. Rush, according to the internet, died in June, 2013.

OF COURSE, THE spay clinics that originated in California, or elsewhere, were not welcome news to the nation's veterinarians, any more than was our clinic in Oklahoma fifteen to twenty years later.

One independent thinker, Dr. Lloyd Faulkner, a veterinarian at Colorado State University, however, understood the pet overpopulation problem—even back in 1971. He wrote an article entitled "Spay Clinics," that was published in the Autumn 1971 *American Animal Hospital Association Bulletin.*

I have quoted Dr. Faulkner from that article, epigraphically, and extensively, in numerous chapters of this book. I have not, to this date, read anything more compelling, with regard to the great divide between veterinarians and humanitarians, on the subject of pet overpopulation. It is important to emphasize the date it was written. Autumn 1971. Forty-nine years ago.

Dr. Faulkner admonished his colleagues, back then, to take the overpopulation of dogs and cats seriously, and do whatever possible to resolve it: "We are an hour late and a dollar short in our desire to discover the mechanisms of reproduction in dogs and cats and in the development of technologies to control the process. We are tardy in enlisting the capabilities of the profession in support of the cause of the humanists."

The veterinarians were, back in 1971, an hour late and a dollar short in the battle against pet overpopulation. They are, forty-nine years, and millions—or billions—of dead dogs and cats, late in 2020.

Forty-nine years and counting.

Dr. Lloyd Faulker. My hero. A veterinarian. He gave it his best shot.

I learned Dr. Faulker had retired, and was living in Stillwater, Oklahoma. Sometime around 2002, some thirty years after his article was published, I placed a call to him.

I introduced myself, and told him how I had, for years, kept a copy of his article.

"I want to tell you how right on you were then, and continue to be now," I said. I told him I had distributed copies of the article to dozens of veterinarians and organizations throughout the years.

The first words out of his mouth were, "Not much has changed, has it?"

We continued to speak about the pet overpopulation tragedy, and the failure of veterinarians throughout the years to recognize their role in resolving it.

I ended our conversation by profusely thanking him again for his futile efforts to lead a blind profession out of the darkness.

DR. MARVIN MACKIE, another savvy neuter/spay pioneer, opened his first neuter/spay clinic in California in 1976, the first of four, that were called Animal Birth Control Clinics. When we named our clinic that same name in 1985, we had no clue the clinics existed in California.

In a phone conversation, Dr. Mackie, like Dr. Faulkner, expressed his disappointment with the veterinary community for its position on spay clinics, calling it "a professional embarrassment."

Dr. Mackie recommends, however, those who face veterinary opposition, when establishing spay clinics, continue with their plans, because, he says, the veterinary community knows they are fighting a losing battle.

Right on, Dr. Mackie.

CHAPTER 15

"We know that a shelter work . . . is not merely a matter of sentiment, though I may say . . . God help the world if there were no sentiment in man: or, I would better say, that God does help the suffering of the world through sentiment implanted in man: and when we are striving against sentiment, by which I mean noble and tender feeling, we are striving against God." — Mrs. Huntington Smith, founder of the Animal Rescue League of Boston, 1899

Please find enclosed our bid for operation of the Lawton Animal Shelter, along with the requested documents, as well as other documents pertinent to the operation of an animal shelter.

As pointed out in the past few months, those of us concerned with conditions at the current city operated animal shelter believe that a shelter should make a positive contribution to the community and in turn receive community support.

If the Humane Society should prove to be the successful bidder, we will make every effort to improve the general image of the shelter as (a) a humane, safe place for stray or unwanted animals to be taken, (b) a place where the public can adopt healthy pets, and (c) a place where the public is welcome and will be treated courteously, properly assisted, and appreciated.

We've come through a long, drawn out process in pursuit of a more humane animal shelter. We're now presenting our best effort to you. Fate will determine the outcome.

ABOVE ARE EXCERPTS from a letter I, representing the newly formed Lawton Animal Sheltering Committee, wrote to Mayor Wayne Gilley and members of the Lawton City Council, dated October 7, 1986—less than seventeen months after the Animal Birth Control Clinic opened its doors.

ACCOUNTS OF THE deplorable conditions that existed at our local animal control facility were reaching us more and more frequently via Animal

Birth Control Clinic customers and pet owners. We were the only humane game in town and, if it concerned animal welfare in a hundred-mile radius, it was brought to our attention.

Both animal control and the animal shelter were operated out of the police department. The animal control officers, who were all men (and not necessarily men who were kind to animals), were in charge of everything. Each year, they rounded up the strays, tossed food into the cages, and handled about a thousand adoptions and reclaims. The six or seven thousand "leftovers," that no one claimed or wanted, were euthanized and hauled to the municipal landfill. According to animal control statistics, in 1984, officers also retrieved 3,900 dead animals from Lawton streets.

I avoided the local animal shelter like the plague. But, for some reason that I fail to recall, I had occasion to go there alone, once, possibly to pick up some shelter statistics I had requested. One particular dog drew my attention. It was a very old white Poodle. The dog's eyes were cloudy and matted, but what disturbed me most was that it was trembling uncontrollably with fear.

As I write this today, it sickens me that I didn't take that dog home with me. I am sure it was because I already had too many dogs; and that was before I could face euthanasia. But I would do it today, even if it meant it would have to be euthanized; because I could give it the comfort and love it was desperately needing, and it would no longer be afraid in the last days of its life.

It turns out the white Poodle is just one layer, of hundreds of layers, of emotional baggage I would carry for a lifetime, as a result of this ofttimes, seemingly God-forsaken cause I chose for myself, or somehow was chosen for me.

I PERSONALLY WOULD receive phone calls at home, and at the car dealership, from concerned citizens describing the conditions they had seen at the animal shelter, such as the hose cleaning of cages, without first removing litters of puppies and kittens.

One evening, I received one of those calls as I was sitting down to dinner with my family.

I didn't know the caller. He sounded like a young man who was almost ready to break into tears. "Mrs. Delluomo. That man just hosed those baby kittens down, and walked away, and left them soaking wet. It was so pitiful. Something has to be done."

I immediately called the chief-of-police at his home, and at his dinner time. If my dinner was to be ruined by these calls, regarding the deficiencies of his department, then, by damned, so was his.

On any one of these calls, I would be assured those practices would be eliminated. They were not.

IF I HAVE left the impression that all was going well at the ABC Clinic, and we had time on our hands to embroil ourselves in more controversy, then I have badly misinformed. To say, rather, that we were working our tails off was putting it mildly.

In those days, we were paranoid about the work we were doing. We knew we were operating under a microscope (pun intended). We kept surgery animals two nights to be sure they were properly fasted before surgery and could be watched closely after surgery. The clinic closed at 5:30 p.m. each surgery day, and volunteers went in around 10:00 p.m. to check on the animals.

Like most human surgeries, these days neuters and spays are performed on an outpatient basis. Animals go home the same day of surgery, except in rare cases where the doctor wants an animal kept over, or a red-neck pet owner won't agree to keep an outside dog or cat indoors for a couple of days.

Clinic finances were disturbing, to say the least. Like any new business, we were struggling. However, we were not like any new business. We were a nonprofit with rock bottom prices, and a bylaw in our constitution that stated no pet owner would be turned away regardless of his or her ability to pay. That was a tough row to hoe.

If the task of the clinic paper work and finances had fallen on my shoulders, there might not be a clinic today. My paid bills and receipts go into one of the small plastic tubs, and months later, I may, grudgingly, get them properly filed.

Linda was wrangling with those tasks, while putting in eight hours on the job at Prudential. On a daily basis, she would stop by the clinic, pick up paper work, go to the bank, take the daily ledger home with her for scrutiny, and then forward everything to the accountant in order to keep us straight with the IRS. As clinic administrator, she does all that, and more, to this day.

She took the finances personal. I can't count the times she called me literally in tears.

"I don't know what we're going to do," she would wail. "We owe Pfizer five thousand dollars and we've got two thousand dollars in the bank.

I would do my best to console her. "We'll just do what we have to do."

Of course, that meant put in our own money, call people who we knew would be good for a quick hundred bucks, and then plan another garage sale.

Our fund-raising included such escapades as setting up booths and selling homemade ice cream at the local Arts for All and International Arts Festivals. We placed funny-looking plastic dog banks in local businesses for donations. But, perhaps—no, not perhaps—for sure, our most bizarre fund-raising effort of all was operating a bingo hall.

Did I just say that? Did I just say we operated a bingo hall? Well, yes we did. And most of us weren't even Catholic.

I have to admit that venture was not very profitable. The money my husband had loaned the organization to buy into that business was never repaid, and the fact that we had no idea what the hell we were doing didn't help either.

But we tried it, and that was that.

Oh, I don't know. Maybe we would have run a whore house if we could have been assured it would have stopped the suffering and senseless killing of an excess of unwanted dogs and cats.

But, probably, the last thing in the world we needed to do was take over the operation of the City of Lawton Animal Shelter, and get smack dab in the middle of another fight with—you know—the Comanche County Veterinary Medical Association!

CHAPTER 16

"Far better it is to dare mighty things, to win glorious triumphs even though checkered by failure, than to rank with those poor spirits who neither enjoy nor suffer much because they live in the gray twilight that knows neither victory nor defeat." — Theodore Roosevelt

I UNDERSTAND WHY the National Rifle Association goes into a frenzy at the mere whisper of gun regulation. The proliferation of guns is beneficial in terms of power and money. I get that.

The same is true of the American Kennel Club. I understand that when hundreds of thousands of litters of purebred puppies are born, and then registered each year with the AKC, the trips to the bank are frequent.

And yes, you read that right. That's hundreds of thousands of litters of puppies produced by AKC breeders each and every year. Then, when those puppies are sold, each have to be registered as individual dogs. Then, often, those dogs grow up and produce another round of litters that, in turn, need to be registered. Then more trips to the bank. And then . . . well, you get the picture.

I understand this. It's money. It's power. It's politics. I totally get it. I don't like it. But I get it. And I think I might be able to muster up at least a scintilla of sympathy or understanding of the veterinarian position on spay clinics and low-cost neuter/spay programs. The competition may very well impact the full service clinic's bottom line.

So there you have it. I have graciously conceded that, most likely, low-cost spay clinics may have at least some detrimental financial effect on full service veterinary clinics.

But I have never known a single animal advocate to request the veterinary community lower their prices on any other surgical procedure, teeth cleaning, x-rays or general care. Linda just paid $3,500 for cataract surgery for her granddog. When I shell out $175 to $200 for one of my dog's teeth cleaning, I don't complain—although it is more than it costs to have my teeth cleaned. My daughter's friend, who is a paraplegic, is saving money from his paycheck for knee surgery for his dog. The quoted price for the surgery: $3,000. No one is complaining. No one, that I can name, has asked veterinarians to reduce their prices for any other procedures, other than neutering and spaying.

Pardon me for saying it yet again. Dogs and cats are dying. The number one cause of death in dogs and cats in America is euthanasia; not parvo or distemper; not leptospirosis, feline leukemia, rhinotracheitis, caliciviris, panleukopenia, or any other multiple syllable disease. In the absence of safe and painless nonsurgical sterilization procedures, and restrictive breeding laws, low- cost neuters and spays are crucial. It is a moral, not an economic, issue. It's all we have.

The veterinarians, however, feel humane societies are infringing on their turf. And if the opposition we in Lawton, and others, have experienced from veterinarians was limited only to the subject of low-cost neuter/spay programs, this book might never have been written.

But, regretfully, that has not been the case.

It was becoming obvious if we wanted to live in a humane community, something would have to be done about the animal shelter. There was not one good thing that anyone in town could say about it. That is, except for most of the local veterinarians, and the local newspaper.

City council members were also getting complaints about the conditions at the animal shelter. I had begun telling those who were calling me to contact their representatives. We instructed clinic employees to do the same.

We had heard about other communities forming humane societies and taking over their municipal shelters under contract with their cities. Waco, Texas, had done just that—successfully.

The old shelter building was deplorable, with a metal roof that intensified the hot Oklahoma sun in summer; where rain poured in by the bucketfuls; and rats, the size of small kittens, called the place home.

Unfortunately, this description of Lawton's animal shelter back in the eighties is true of hundreds of animal shelters to this day.

To the police department's credit, they had requested a new building and it had been approved. But no one really believed that care of the animals would significantly improve. While rain would no longer leak into the kennels, it was doubtful that new construction would suddenly instill compassion in the hearts of the animals' caretakers.

July and August in Oklahoma can reach temperatures of 110 degrees, or higher, and rumors were that the dogs were locked in that metal-roofed building on weekends with no air conditioning, and no one went in to feed or water them.

"WHY DON'T YOU just go out there and picket the place?" suggested City Councilman Bob Shanklin, who had become a ringleader on the council for the animal shelter cause.

On an extremely hot Sunday afternoon, armed with a permit for demonstrating and Councilman Shanklin's support, we did just that. An impressive number of concerned citizens showed up, as did KSWO TV. Signs of protest, demanding a more humane animal shelter, waved in the hot Oklahoma sun.

We discovered on that Sunday afternoon, much to our dismay, the rumors of dogs being locked in the oven-like conditions of that dilapidated, metal-roofed building, were indeed true.

The police department got wind of the demonstration, and a couple of animal control officers showed up and opened the building to give the dogs some much-needed ventilation.

WE BEGAN TO have conversations with Waco and other communities where humane societies were operating their city's animal shelter under contract. We visited with most of the council members, except the ones we had heard were unsupportive of our proposal. We left them alone temporarily. We talked to the city manager and the police chief.

What we were proposing was what Waco and others had done to resolve problems with their animal shelter operations.

Toni DeStephano of Wichita Falls was helpful for a second time. The Humane Society of Wichita Falls has historically had an animal sheltering relationship with the City of Wichita Falls. Again, she offered us help and encouragement. She later would help train our shelter employees to perform euthanasia.

At one point, Toni took me aside to give me some advice—advice I didn't want to hear or heed. "Deloris," she said, "you need to become certified to euthanize animals.

What? I was insulted. I was horrified. "There's no way. I never could. I never would."

"Look," she said, "you always need the most compassionate people to do that job."

"That's not why I got into this work," I responded, almost angrily. "Not to kill animals. Besides we're working here to get to a point where euthanasia is not necessary in Lawton."

"How are you going to do that?" she asked.

"Well, you know we're trying to neuter and spay everything in sight. And we're going to get laws that make it tough to breed, or even own, an unaltered dog or cat."

My naivete was totally exposed.

"It will never happen," she said.

Toni was a realist. I was a dreamer. I really believed we could end pet overpopulation. It was a matter of simple math—of supply and demand.

BY NOW WE had the city's attention. Next, we formed the Lawton Animal Sheltering Committee. I am uncertain when the first official request went to the city for a study on our proposal to contract with the City of Lawton to operate the animal shelter. It had to be late March or early April 1986.

No committee meetings or hearings had even been set.

The CCVMA, however, got wind early on of what we were proposing, and, in what had become their trademark knee-jerk reaction, immediately set out to stop us in our tracks!

This, too, doctors? This, too?

CHAPTER 17

"I know at last what distinguishes man from animals: financial worries." — Jomain Roland, French Novelist and Essayist

THE VETERINARIANS' LETTER to Councilman Keith Jackson, with copies to the nine other council members, was dated April 17, 1986, and signed by every veterinarian in Lawton, except for Dr. Carl Manske. I never knew Dr. Manske. Out of curiosity, I called him many years later to inquire as to why he didn't sign. He was fairly noncommittal. To the best of my recollection, he simply said he didn't want to sign, or saw no need. For whatever his reason, I have always been grateful.

The letter at least conceded our group was "dedicated to honorable humanitarian work," but "not qualified and should not be involved in city animal control/public health or in the practice of veterinary medicine." The letter referred to us as "self-proclaimed experts."

If they had bothered to check, they would have realized that animal control was to remain in the hands of the police department. Public health, of course, would stay with the health department, and the veterinarians who worked for us would continue to practice veterinary medicine by neutering and spaying dogs and cats. We wanted to take care of homeless animals and we certainly were qualified to do that!

In their letter, the vets offered a treatise on rabies and other zoonotic diseases, and elaborated on how a "buffer zone" must be created to protect humans and wildlife—that buffer zone being vaccination of our household pets and, "removing stray animals from the streets."

The veterinarians praised the animal control wardens as "professionals in their field." The letter spoke of the outstanding rapport between personnel at the animal shelter and local veterinarians, with the common goal of protecting the public from rabies and other zoonotic diseases. They played up that "zoonotic" disease thing a lot, but I don't recall ever having an outbreak of anything here—at least where dogs and cats are concerned.

How nice it would have been if local veterinarians could have simply formed an outstanding rapport with a local humane organization, sharing the common goal of neutering and spaying dogs and cats to protect them from death caused by pet overpopulation. Could they have just talked to us?

We never wanted this war. What was it with these people?

Toward the end of the letter, they got to the real heart of the matter: "The CCVMA feels certain that if LUV-ABC obtains operation of the Animal Shelter, they will establish a full service veterinary clinic in said facility. Since LUV-ABC is a tax exempt organization, this would constitute unfair competition with local and area veterinarians. Operations such as this have been declared unlawful by the Supreme Courts of Michigan and Virginia. The Animal Birth Control Clinic, currently operated by LUV-ABC, is in violation of the Oklahoma Veterinary Practice Act and efforts are underway by the Oklahoma State Board of Veterinary Medical Examiners to stop this situation."

The veterinarians were wrong! We had no intentions of establishing a full service veterinary clinic in said facility. And we already had a spay clinic. Why would we need another one? Besides, they said themselves that efforts were underway by the Oklahoma State Board of Veterinary Medical Examiners to "stop this situation." What did they have to fear?

"The CCVMA urges the City of Lawton," the letter continued, "in the strongest of terms, to maintain control and operation of the Animal Shelter just as it is at the present time."

Just as it is? Keep the shelter just as it is?

If the veterinarians believed Lawton was running a humane animal shelter at that time, they were a very small percentage of the 100,000 people in Lawton and Fort Sill who thought so—except for editors at the local newspaper.

Shortly after council members received the letter from the CCVMA, an op-ed appeared in the Sunday, May 3, 1986, newspaper in support of the veterinarians' position.

The first paragraph read: "A proposal to transfer control of the city animal shelter from the City to a group of local citizens is lacking in real merit and should be rejected if and when it is presented to the City Council."

The editorial stated that the proposal, "being packaged by Deloris Delluomo of the shelter society," was opposed by a group of fifteen veterinarians who had drafted a letter to council members . . . "This came in response to a Delluomo campaign to enlist individual council support before it is presented to the governing body."

Oh, so now it was unethical for citizens to speak to their council representatives outside the total "governing body"?

The paper warned of escalating costs if "the society gains control of the shelter. We doubt if the taxpayers would be willing to boost animal shelter costs merely to assuage some local animal lovers while compromising the real goals of an animal shelter."

And just what exactly was their description of the real goals of an animal shelter?

The article ended with this: "Humane society contributions to animal welfare are well known, but we believe the city-operated animal shelter is doing a good job and should be left alone."

As was the case with the veterinarians' letter to council members, much of what the newspaper had to say was inaccurate. No one had talked to any one of us. Perhaps the writer of the editorial should have taken the calls the clinic was receiving, and I was getting at home, or letters that were being written by citizens, with regard to the conditions at the "tax-supported" animal shelter.

And just why was I always singled out for criticism? Many people in Lawton supported what we were trying to do. The Lawton Animal Sheltering Committee was comprised of fifteen reputable Lawtonians, ranging in diversity from an interior designer to a Merrill Lynch stockbroker, and a retired military officer.

As quickly as I heard about the CCVMA letter, I, representing our committee, wrote a letter to Councilman Jackson, and the other members of the council.

"It is not difficult to understand why the local veterinarians object to the work of the Lawton United Volunteers for Animal Birth Control because, from their viewpoint, our high-quality, low-cost neuter/spay facility is hurting their business," our letter stated. "We are able to prove, however, that a large percentage of the over 1500 pet owners who have used the Animal Birth Control Clinic, since it opened 11 months ago, would never have been able to use the neuter/spay services of the higher priced veterinarians. Therefore, those animals would still be producing litter after litter of unwanted puppies and kittens that, ultimately, would have to be dealt with by the city and the taxpayer."

What was so hard to understand? If more dogs and cats were neutered and spayed, less puppies and kittens would be born. And if less puppies and kittens were born, then less money and human resources would have to be spent on animal control and killing animals. And if less money and human resources were spent on animal control and killing animals, there would then be a great savings to taxpayers all over the kingdom. And everyone would live happily ever after.

My letter pointed out that "those of us involved in humane work and animal welfare causes are overworked and underpaid as it is (as a matter of fact, we are not paid at all.) For those veterinarians to assume that we need to volunteer more of our time and money to establish and operate a full-service veterinary clinic is not only absurd, but almost laughable."

MY OLD WEBSTER'S Dictionary describes veterinary as "the branch of medicine dealing with the prevention and treatment of diseases and injuries in animals, esp. domestic animals."

Wouldn't a bottle of sodium pentobarbital, the death solution used for euthanasia, pose the most serious threat of all to the domestic animal, as far as veterinary medicine is concerned?

What is it that cartloads of dead animals, or incinerated ashes at municipal landfills, bring to veterinarians' practices that they so desperately want to preserve?

CHAPTER 18

"There is nothing more frightful than ignorance in action." — Johann Wolfgang von Goethe, German writer

"THIS IS A dog pound, which is a place like a jail," said Dr. Dan Woesner, member of the CCVMA. "We don't call our jail a criminal shelter. That is what this is because any animal going in there is violating the law by running loose if for no other reason. For this reason, the desires of the humane society is at cross purposes with the desires of the pound."

Dr. Woesner, a doctor of animals, actually said that.

He said the unfortunate homeless dogs and cats that wind up in animal shelters were criminals and deserved the death penalty?

No. He was unequivocally wrong. The uncaring, irresponsible humans, to whom those poor innocent creatures once belonged, are the criminals. They are the ones who deserve to be in jail. For every pet who ends up as a stray on the road, or in an animal shelter, there is a breeder or pet owner who is responsible for that dog or cat being in that situation.

This brings to mind a commentary written years ago by syndicated columnist Andy Rooney, about his friend, writer, and journalist Cleveland Amory, who was an animal rights activist.

"An open season on hunters is an idea suggested by Cleveland Amory as a way of keeping down the growing number of hunters in this country," Rooney wrote. "Amory insists he is only thinking of what is best for the hunters themselves when he suggests that some of them should be harvested every year.

"If their ranks are not thinned out, he says, they'll become so numerous that food supplies for them will be inadequate and many of them will die of starvation.

"Hunters have become so numerous, Amory says, that they are a nuisance in many areas. Hunters are often seen loose, invading back yards and gardens in residential areas, having been forced out of the woods by their own numbers.

"Amory wants the hunting of hunters to be carried out in a civilized way. For instance, if someone bags a hunter, Amory does feel that the dead hunter should be tied to the roof or hood of the hunter's car when being brought back from where it was shot."

Oh, of course, we in a civilized society, would never think of "bagging" hunters. Nor would we ever suggest euthanizing irresponsible pet owners and breeders, just because there are too many of them. We only do that to the innocent animals they bring into the world; the ones someone abandons on a desolate back road because they are no longer wanted; or the ones who sit, quivering in fear, in, both humane and inhumane, tax-supported animal shelters, waiting to die—while breeders and irresponsible pet owners walk away scot free.

Dr. Woesner, the veterinarian, said all those things about stray animals being criminals; and he said much, much more. It's right there in the minutes of the committee meeting held at city hall on July 1, 1986, at 5:15 p.m.

The mayor and city council had established the eight-member committee at the council meeting on June 10, 1986, upon tabling an agenda item to consider our proposal to operate the Lawton animal shelter under contract with the city. Our proposal would have to be studied.

In addition to Dr. Woesner, other appointed members were present, including the chief of police, and the director of the Comanche County Health Department.

Councilman Keith Jackson was appointed to chair the committee.

Dr. Woesner, who was the foremost opponent of the proposal, made his feelings known on every subject discussed. Not only did he believe homeless pets were law violators, he didn't believe there was any scenario wherein they should be adopted. He spoke against "adoption under any system by anyone."

"I would advise anyone not to go down, take out a stray animal, and take it into your home," Woesner said.

He was one of those veterinarians who advocated letting a pet have at least one litter, but he didn't believe in shelter adoptions that would, ultimately, be a result of those first litters.

He explained that cats are carriers of toxoplasmosis, which is shed in their stools. He warned that if a "stray animal defecates in a yard and a woman is pregnant and digs in the garden with her bare hands" she can pick that up and it can cause birth defects, abortion, and many other diseases. Furthermore, he said, there is no way anyone can guarantee that a stray cat is not a carrier of toxoplasmosis without exhaustive tests.

I knew enough about toxoplasmosis to, at least, ask some pertinent questions. When my daughter-in-law was pregnant, I had been curious about the disease at that time because I had cats in my home.

I posed what I thought to be a somewhat tricky question to Dr. Woesner: "Doctor, isn't it true that someone's seemingly healthy cat who lives in his or her home, and sleeps on his or her bed, could also carry toxoplasmosis? It doesn't have to be a stray, does it?"

I continued on before he had a chance to answer. "If there is a healthy cat in the house, that cat can be a carrier . . . even though it isn't a stray. Right?"

He used a weird analogy to explain: "Well, I don't think you would be as afraid to kiss your husband as you would be to kiss a stranger down on First Street."

Huh? What?

Dr. Woesner distributed six pages of his handwritten recommendations to committee members, itemizing his objections to our proposal. He wrote: "Strays are law violators just like speeders, etc; strays are potential disease carriers, and majority need (he underlined the word need) to be euthanized; strays knock over and scatter garbage, encouraging flys, roaches, mice, rats, etc."

Yeah. Looking for a crumb of food.

Was there anything Dr. Woesner liked about animals?

What was really troubling to me is that I had used this veterinarian for my own animals several times in the past. I remember one particular incident, where my youngest son was bitten by a small, stray kitten in our front yard. This took place at our home that was located within the city limits, before the move to the country, and before I was involved in animal causes. Inasmuch as we were going on a family vacation to visit my sister in Hawaii, I left the cat to be quarantined with Dr. Woesner. I didn't know then what I would come to know later. As far as I could tell, the cat was healthy and I am not so sure that my seven-year-old son didn't provoke the bite.

After a few days, I called Dr. Woesner from Hawaii, only to learn that the cat had died. Died of what? I don't even recall the reason he gave as I was a bit panicked about the welfare of my son. He advised me he had sent the head off to a laboratory for rabies testing.

As I look back, I can't help but wonder if this was one of those strays that Dr. Woesner thought needed to be euthanized. He also euthanized Jacklyn, our first family dog, that we thought had cancer. I, and others in our group, had actually used this person to care for our pets before we learned the truth about him. He didn't try to talk me out of euthanizing my dog, and I allowed him to take her to the back of his clinic, without me there, something I would never do today. I was naive, and I still, to this day, pay for my ignorance with those layers and layers of emotional baggage. I only hope that Jacklyn and that kitten are in a good place, and have forgiven me.

WHEN IT COMES to character failings, I am as flawed as any average Jane on the planet. I am extremely impatient, I have the tenacity of a pit bull's jaw, and I cuss like a sailor. Throughout the years of battling veterinarians and others for the cause of animal welfare, however, I have understood it is imperative that I maintain as high a level of integrity and credibility as is humanly possible. I have been sure to do my homework with regard to programs we were pursuing, and changes in policies we were advocating.

I remained calm in spite of Dr. Woesner's nonsense. There was no need for me to try and discredit him. He was doing a good job of that by himself.

I did my best to answer questions asked by Councilman Jackson and others on the committee. I had been talking to Waco on a regular basis to learn all I could about their program. In fact, I felt like I had newly made friends in Waco. Members of their humane society had even been to Lawton to visit the Animal Birth Control Clinic in anticipation of building their own clinic.

I had obtained copies of an International City Management Association report entitled "Management Information Service Report," which I distributed to members of the committee. The entire report dealt with animal control and indicated that a good licensing ordinance can bring needed revenue into a city.

I pointed out that we planned on proposing better licensing ordinances in the city.

Dr. Woesner was unyielding in his opposition to dog and cat licensing (what wasn't he opposed to?) even though much of his oppositional rhetoric to our shelter proposal had been city budgetary concerns. "A wise city council eliminated the unfair discriminatory tax on dogs and cats years ago," he wrote in his recommendations. "People appreciated . . . Taxing personal property is dangerous precedent. Might lead to taxing children, or boats or car dealers cars or anything else an irresponsible council might think of."

Remember Sue Neal who was at that first meeting at my house? She is the lady who currently lives near Tyler, Texas, and deals with strays unceasingly? Her late husband at that time was a local boat dealer and, of course, my husband was a car dealer. Is there a remote possibility that Dr. Woesner could have been referring to our husbands in the above statement concerning the licensing of dogs and cats?

Do you get the connection? I didn't either.

I suggested to the committee that, as a non-profit organization, we could solicit donations for additional income, something the City could not very well do. I informed the committee that we expected to have a good working relationship with animal control officers.

With regard to Woesner's obvious dislike and fear of stray animals, I told the committee that I had personally picked up countless numbers of strays over the years, including pit bulls on chains, and had been bitten only once—by a Chihuahua.

Trying not to appear argumentative, I did, however, tell Dr. Woesner I believed his talk about toxoplasmosis was nothing more than a scare tactic.

"I don't think so," he said.

To his credit, Councilman Jackson interrupted this back and forth. "I like to live in the reality, and realistically I do not visualize ever stopping the adoption process."

Thank you, Mr. Jackson, for drawing the discussion back from the edge of insanity.

CHAPTER 19

"Would you want to adopt an animal from the shelter only to watch
it suffer, really suffer, and then die? I was told each time I adopted my
dogs that if they were sick, to bring them back and get another one.
That's expected when buying a piece of clothing, not when adopting an
animal to join your family." — Gwyn Smith, Lawton citizen, in a May
9, 1986, letter to City Manager Robert Metzinger

SUPPORT WAS STRONG among citizens for an improved city animal
shelter. On May 9, 1986, Mrs. Gwyn Smith wrote a letter to City Manager
Robert Metzinger with carbon copies to Mayor Wayne Gilley, Councilman Mel
Fredricksen, and to us.

Mrs. Smith's impassioned letter described her experience of adopting two
dogs from the animal shelter, both of which had died, one of distemper and one
of parvo, and the emotional devastation she had experienced.

"When I explained to a shelter employee . . . the cost of trying to save the first
dog, his statement was: "that was stupid to spend that much money on a dog.
Not what you would expect to hear from an animal shelter employee," she wrote.

She explained that her concern was "not necessarily the expense," but the fact
that the animals receive no medical care when they fall ill.

"Also," Mrs. Smith wrote, "it is my understanding that food is tossed into the
cages and only the bigger and stronger animals get to eat, while the smaller or
sick animals starve. This feeding practice was witnessed by a friend many times."

Her letter stated: "I honestly believe the citizens of this City would be more
receptive to the shelter if they knew the City of Lawton and the shelter employees
were doing more to protect and care for these animals and were working to rid
the City of distemper and parvo."

Her letter exhibited her passion for her pets that had just died. She made
recommendations to the city as to what she believed citizens want in their animal
shelter: "I honestly believe that the shelter could and should purchase the proper
vaccine for distemper and parvo and inoculate each and every animal brought
into the shelter. Also, that each animal should be kept in a separate enclosure for
a certain time period before being put into the general animal population."

She pointed out that she believed people would be willing to pay extra for adoptions if each animal was immunized and free of disease.

"You can see what is happening at the shelter and the strong need to make changes and prevent the spread of disease and suffering of the many animals brought there. I have heard from so many, many, people who will not go to the shelter to adopt because of the conditions there, which only leads to the increased number of adoptable animals put to death."

Mrs. Smith ended her letter with a passionate plea for the city to consider the "need for action and reform in the care and handling of these innocent animals" and to put a stop to all the "needless suffering and at the same time try to reduce the cases of parvo and distemper in our City."

This is the animal shelter Lawton veterinarians said, "in the strongest of terms," should remain under the control and operation of the city "just as it is at the present time."

This is the animal shelter the local newspaper said "is doing a good job and should be left alone."

This is the animal shelter that, years later, would be back in that same condition, or worse.

OUR BATTLES WITH the veterinarians continued over the next few months as we struggled to gain the support of council members and city officials. The local newspaper had early on proven they were not in our camp.

In addition to local support, many others, however, beyond the city limits, were strong supporters of humanely operated animal shelters.

On May 16, 1986, Mr. John Hatchel, Deputy City Manager of the City of Waco, wrote a letter to Assistant City Manager Melissa Vossmer. He praised his City's decision to contract with their local humane society. He ended his letter with this: "As you can tell, we are quite pleased with this working arrangement and think it is providing a better service for our citizens."

On May 27, 1986, State Senator Billie Floyd wrote a letter to City Manager Robert Metzinger, detailing how she and a group of citizens in Ada, Oklahoma, "helped work with this kind of agreement for the City of Ada and our Pontotoc County Animal Welfare Shelters. I think that this agreement has been very beneficial for the City of Ada, the animal control officers and the Humane Shelter, not to mention the animals."

Senator Floyd wrote: "I would recommend that you check into the possibility of allowing the Humane Society to operate their shelter." She offered her assistance and added that she was very active in the program in Ada.

On June 4, 1986, Barbara Cassidy, Director of Animal Sheltering and Control of the Humane Society of the United States wrote a letter to Mr. Metzinger supporting our proposal. "Although there are no firm national statistics on the number of contract operations in the U.S., our surveys and direct contact with shelters across the country indicate that there are approximately 50% shelters operating on a contractual basis. In the immediate Washington D.C. area, there are no fewer than five contractual operations, several of which have been in existence for over 20 years. The Washington D.C. animal control facility and spay/neuter clinic are successfully operated by the Washington Humane Society."

Ms. Cassidy wrote that HSUS believes that the "community animal control program is a municipal responsibility, however, contracting with a local humane society is a viable alternative, that, when adequately funded by the local government, can meet the community's needs."

This was not the first letter we had received from HSUS. Early on, we had received a letter from Patrick Parkes, Vice President of Field Services, commending us on our work at the Animal Birth Control Clinic in the battle against pet overpopulation.

There would be other letters from other officers at HSUS and other organizations, far and away from Lawton, concerning the work we were doing here.

PERHAPS I AM out of line for suggesting it, but whoever treated Mrs. Smith's adopted dogs did make for themselves a nice little profit—even though both dogs died. And what Mrs. Smith would probably have had a difficult time even comprehending is that her own veterinarian—whoever it was—would, most likely, have opposed vaccinating shelter animals against parvo and distemper.

When it became obvious that the City was in support of our proposal, and a contract had been drawn up, a memorandum on the City of Lawton letterhead was sent to all council members dated September 9, 1986, from Councilman Mel Fredricksen requesting "serious consideration be given to making the attached changes to the animal sheltering agreement." The veterinarians' attorney (now they had an attorney?) submitted the request for the changes.

The first request was to add the following to Page 4 of the contract: "The City Manager may establish from time to time appropriate rules and regulations setting forth the maximum time any animal may be held prior to manditory (sic) destruction."

The veterinarians had voiced concerns that because we were "animal lovers," the shelter and town would be overrun with strays. They wanted assurance that an animal was not allowed to live past its expiration date—that, God forbid, any homeless, abandoned, unwanted dog or cat received one more day of life than it truly or legally deserved.

The most significant request made by Lawton veterinarians was that the following language be added to Page 27.01. Item #28: A. Services. No vaccinations, spay, neuter, worming, discretionary veterinary service shall be permitted to be performed by the lessee.

B. Advertisement. No advertising of any veterinarian, clinic, or organization shall be permitted on the premises either by written or verbal recommendation by any contractor, agent or employee.

Now just what is the definition of paranoia?

Let me see if I can describe it.

Any pet owner, although it is never recommended, can go to the farmers co-op and buy vaccinations and worming medicine for their pets. But the veterinarians wanted to prevent the humane society from vaccinating or de-worming pets that had been turned over to us and were now legally owned by us—even if worms were flowing out their rear ends. And they wanted to prevent us from having pets neutered or spayed before adoption, even though that was actually a state law for adopted pets from animal shelters even back then.

Obviously, the majority of council members saw right through this paranoia. The veterinarians lost on all points, and the proposal stood as drafted.

Now let's look at the real reason Mrs. Smith, who I don't recall ever having met, and other citizens, were having such a hard time adopting healthy animals from the City of Lawton animal shelter.

It can be summed up in one word. Veterinarians.

CHAPTER 20

"I care not for a man's religion whose dog and cat are not the better for it." — Abraham Lincoln

"CITY HUMANE GROUP wins shelter bid."

That was the headline in the Wednesday, October 15, 1986, edition of the Lawton Morning Press. Yes, we got control of the city animal shelter. The task that lay ahead was monumental. That old saying "Be careful what you wish for" flashed across my mind.

"A weary Lawton City Council awarded a contract for the operation of the city's animal control shelter to the Humane Society of Lawton-Comanche County at Tuesday's meeting," wrote Kim McConnell, staff writer for the newspaper.

"The action came after council members spent two hours discussing a motion to terminate City Manager Robert Metzinger . . . and the shelter contract was approved with no discussion, with council members Mel Fredericksen, Leila Barfield and Bill Scearce voting against the measure."

Council members Bob Shanklin, Frank Walker, Red Miller, Gene Love, Keith Jackson, Jeff Irwin and Coleman Johnson voted for a more humane animal shelter for the City of Lawton.

I don't recall why the city manager was fired, but it had nothing to do with us or our proposal. We had formed a humane society just weeks before, when it was almost certain our proposal was going to be approved. We now had two non-profit designations to keep up with: The Lawton United Volunteers for Animal Birth Control, and The Humane Society of Lawton-Comanche County. An animal shelter and a high volume veterinary surgical facility. Were we nuts?

The paper stated that we submitted the only bid, which was for the ridiculously small sum of $30,500, for operations from Nov. 3 through June 30, the end of the fiscal year. We knew our bid was low, but it was the only possible way to get the animal shelter out of the hands of the police department. And, yes, to the question in the last paragraph.

We had our work cut out for us. For months, we had been searching for an executive director for the shelter. Between the council approval of our contract and the date we were to take possession of the shelter, we hired a director from Texas with experience in animal shelter management.

In the meantime, the city had approved the new shelter facility, and work had been started. We took our husbands to the shelter to paint and perform other manly tasks. We asked citizens to donate funds to help finish the shelter kennels. We asked for bedding, washers and dryers, good quality dog and cat food—all items that were completely foreign to the previous regime.

Believing somehow we could change the world, and perhaps a brick short of a load, we found ourselves knee deep in the shelter business—and all the heartache that goes with it.

SINCE THE NEW shelter was not ready for occupancy, we were forced to operate out of the old building, and we were learning, firsthand, about the rats and the leaking roof.

Late one evening, a heavy downfall of rain had us scrambling to figure out how to get the dogs off a rain-soaked cement floor. And the cats, in their pitiful small facility, were not faring much better.

Mary Evans and Helen Tedder took matters into their own hands. Both elderly women had strong minds of their own and huge hearts for animals. Mary was a retired Major from the U. S. Army, and Helen was a cantankerous, yet much beloved woman, who spent the last years of her life tending to Lawton's thousands of street cats.

Mary and Helen took to the streets on this dark, rainy night, and came back with their station wagons loaded to the hilt with wooden pallets and milk crates.

We were thrilled to behold these treasures they had bestowed on us, as now we could get the animals out of the water.

"Did you get permission to get these?" we asked the ladies.

"No!" they said defiantly—in unison.

Now I think the statute of limitations, for crimes of taking things from back alleys after dark, probably ran out years ago. But Mary and Helen are forever safe from any repercussions anyway, as they both have since gone to be with their Maker.

And there's no way I can know this for sure, but if I were guessing, I would bet the first thing He said to both of them was: "Well done, girls, well done."

Actually, I suspect those wooden pallets and milk crates, that were such life savers for us, and those condemned dogs and cats, were probably in those alleys for disposal, and no crime was committed after all. We'll never know.

I WAS, IN no way, prepared for this job—mentally, emotionally, physically, or financially. The number of beautiful dogs and cats that were brought into that facility on a daily basis were staggering. They arrived either by impoundment by animal control or by citizens who just didn't want them any longer.

I think, probably, when one finds oneself in this type of cause, or any social cause for that matter, both the best and the worst of humanity can be seen.

We had seen the best with the donations and encouragement we were receiving from Lawton citizens, and with the response of pet owners having their dogs and cats neutered and spayed.

Unfortunately, we were about to see the worst.

Although there were literally thousands of heartbreaking situations wherein both dogs and cats ended their lives unwanted in an animal shelter, two dogs come to my mind all these years later. One was a purebred German Shepherd and the other a small Lhasa Apso.

The German Shepherd's owner brought him in. He was neutered and seemed healthy. He was obedience trained and his owner walked him on a leash into the chain-link kennel with dogs barking all around, commanded him to sit and stay, and left him there without so much as a regretful goodbye.

The minister, at the time, of probably the largest protestant denomination in Lawton, brought his family's Lhasa Apso to the front desk. This dog was not well cared for, not groomed, and probably had spent most of its time outdoors. The reverend claimed the family dog had gotten cranky with the children, and gave him up without even a reluctant twinge. Strangely enough, someone who was in the reception area at the time knew the minister, and the dog, and claimed the two small children had harassed and teased the little animal to the point it had probably rebelled.

I agree with Honest Abe. I, too, care not for a man's religion whose dog and cat are not the better for it.

The beautiful German Shepherd and the helpless little Lhasa Apso. Disposable items in a throwaway society. Just two tiny pinpoints on the crowded map of pet overpopulation in America.

BACK IN THE original committee meeting I had told members that we wanted to have a good rapport with animal control officers. That was true. For the sake of animals and citizens alike, it would have been so much better if there had been a combined effort. But they wanted no part of it. They resented the upset of the status quo apple cart and their resentment was palpable.

Their job was to impound animals and enforce the law on the streets and our job was for sheltering only. And, as far as they were concerned, there didn't have to be much dialogue between the two parties to achieve that.

During the Christmas period that year, I left some gifts and cards for each one of them at the front desk. That gesture was never acknowledged.

On another occasion, on one of those 110 degree days in Oklahoma, one of them brought in a red Chow with a litter of tiny puppies. I don't know what the temperature would have been on the metal in the bed of that pickup truck, but it had to be at least 120 degrees. I was outraged to see that nothing had been provided to protect the animals from that torture, but I made every effort to contain my disdain. I asked politely if they would just let me give them a blanket for such occasions. They made it clear that was not my territory and they didn't need my blanket. I think, however, they did finally place a piece of plywood in the back of their trucks—probably because it occurred to them we might decide we wanted to take over animal control and we seemed to be winning all the battles.

WE SETTLED INTO our new job and were considered somewhat of a phenomenon around the state. One of the large TV stations from Oklahoma City flew down in their helicopter to observe this transition from police department to humane society operation.

We were able to adopt a few pets into what we had tried to be sure were good homes but the overwhelming number of animals had no future. We were facing for the first time—for my first time—the dreaded provision of our contract with the City of Lawton: Euthanasia.

Toni DeStephano came up from Wichita Falls that day. I did not involve myself as approximately thirty-five beautiful dogs and cats went to their senseless deaths, and their bodies were carted off on a trailer to the municipal landfill.

I sat outside on a tree stump and sobbed.

CHAPTER 21

"About 30 feet from the door was the incinerator, a thoroughly functional bit of machinery. They wheeled the hamper up to the door, opened it and began throwing corpses onto the heap of gray- black ash. They had a method: each picked up a rear paw and a front paw. They swung the animal forward, then back, then forward again, with a wordless automatic rhythm, the momentum building. On the second swing, at the top of the arc, they released the dead dog, and it flew through the incinerator door with the naturalness of a Michael Jordan free throw." — John Dorschner, "See Spot Die," *The Miami Herald*

FOR YEARS, I have been quoting—with permission—from an article entitled "See Spot Die" written by John Dorschner, a writer for *The Miami Herald*. In the early nineties, Mr. Dorschner embedded himself in the daily activities of the Metro-Dade Animal Services Department, and I personally have never read a more moving account of the daily duties of animal shelter personnel.

Mr. Dorschner details the plight of stray and unwanted animals and animal care workers caught in the never-ending trap of euthanasia—the bottom line result of pet overpopulation.

At that time, according to Dorschner's article, approximately 25,000 dogs and cats were euthanized annually in each of Dade and Broward County.

On one particular day, Dorschner was accompanying Officer John Scally on his rounds. He describes Officer Scally as an animal lover who carries snapshots of his pet Akita. "Single, he coos over the photos as if they were his own offspring," Dorschner reported.

After several stops, Scally and Dorschner responded to a call in a cul-de-sac in Westchester. "A middle-aged woman in a housecoat explained that a mutt had been hanging around her house for days. She had been feeding it, but decided she couldn't care for it any longer," Dorschner wrote.

"The mutt was smallish, dark gray with a furry little beard around the mouth—looking a bit like Tramp in the Disney movie *Lady and the Tramp*.

"Scally slipped a leash on the neck, and Tramp trotted along eagerly to the truck." According to the article, the woman watched Scally lock the dog in the truck and "groaned, realizing the fate that probably awaited the dog. "Aiii. Dios Mio. He hasn't done anything. "Scally filled out the card: 31214-H."

A few days later, Dorschner witnessed the little dog's last moments of life, along with dozens of others who died that day at the Miami Dade Animal Shelter.

"As the dogs arrived, Lily prepared the tray, Dorschner wrote. "It consisted of a half-dozen bottles, each six inches high, filled with a turquoise liquid. On the side was the word POISON, printed in red, flanked by two red skulls and crossbones. Inside was sodium pentobarbital . . . The brand name: Fatal Plus.

"One large dog had so much muscle that it was impossible to find a vein. Lily injected it twice. Still, the dog struggled, breaking loose from Jessica's strong grasp, jumping on the floor.

The dog dashed frantically around for a few moments, then its rear legs collapsed. It rose, took a few steps, collapsed again as the Fatal Plus seeped into its brain," Dorschner wrote.

"With some of the larger dogs, especially the obedient German shepherds, Jessica lifted the front paws up, so that they rested on the table, the rear haunches on the floor. Lily injected the animal, then Jessica tugged at its leash, pulling it off the table, trotting ahead of it five or six steps to the outside door. 'Come on boy. Come on boy,' she said gently. Then swinging open the door and getting another six steps out of the dog, until . . . a few feet away from the incinerator, the dog suddenly stopped, falling over on its side . . . dead! Obedient to the end. Man's best friend . . . Or biggest chump.

"Finally, when only two dogs were left, Jessica picked up the leash of the little bearded guy, the Tramp from the Westchester cul-de-sac. He had been so quiet in the room, but now, at the very last, as Jessica grabbed him and put him on the table, he became suddenly wild, struggling to turn his neck, to get his head away from Jessica.

"But she clasped him firmly. He settled down staring around the room, blinking, waiting. He didn't even flinch when the needle went in. He looked down toward the floor, then off toward the end of the room. And that was it. Thwuppp."

"The girls moved down the hall to the cat room," Dorschner wrote. "There were many cats, but they were quicker work . . . a fast injection into the heart. And after a few minutes, Lily and Jessica had filled a metal shopping cart with dead cats. They lay there, clumps of fur, like so many animal pelts."

Whether it is the Lawton landfill, or the more sophisticated Miami, Florida, incinerator, the killing and disposal of millions of beautiful healthy animals each and every year in this country amounts to a skewed way of thinking—or sheer insanity.

This is America! We can do better than this!

CHAPTER 22

"Mankind's true moral test, its fundamental test (which lies deeply buried from view), consists of its attitude towards those who are at its mercy: animals. And in this respect mankind has suffered a fundamental debacle, a debacle so fundamental that all others stem from it." — Milan Kundera, *The Unbearable Lightness of Being*

OUR CONTRACT TO operate this killing house, commonly referred to as an animal shelter, started on November 3, 1986, and was up for renewal on June 30, 1987.

Job one was killing animals. Oh, we were able to manage a few adoptions, but there was not a snowball's chance in hell that we would ever be able to find homes for the thousands that came into that shelter, year after year. Then there was that stipulation in our contract, insisted on by the veterinarians, that prevented us keeping any pets for an extended period of time. And, even if we could have held pets beyond the designated period, where were we going to put them?

Our very first adoption went awry. The couple that applied for Max the Boxer, appeared to be okay. They answered the questions on the adoption application in a manner that obviously satisfied shelter employees. They even came back a second time to see Max. The rabies coupon came back from the veterinarian. The dog had been rabies vaccinated.

So far, so good.

Max had been adopted on December 17. When the rabies coupon was returned on January 5 and the neuter/spay coupon was not, office manager Deborah Moore became concerned.

A frantic search began. Telephone numbers on the adoption application had been disconnected. Calls to the Ft. Sill military base, and to relatives in Tacoma, Washington, revealed that much of the information on the adoption application had been falsified.

After extensive investigation, Deborah learned that the man on the adoption application was in Germany, but his wife was still in Lawton.

But where was Max?

Thanks to the help of the receptionist at the veterinarian clinic who had redeemed the rabies coupon, Deborah was able to locate the woman who informed her that her husband had taken Max to Washington, and was not planning to have him neutered.

Tammy Lindsay, a humane society board member and adoption follow-up worker, visited the address where the woman supposedly lived in Lawton, and spoke with an older woman who claimed to be the adopter's mother-in-law.

The State of Oklahoma, just two months earlier in November 1986, at the urging of statewide humane advocates—including us—had enacted a state law that required all shelter adoptions be neutered or spayed. The law is still in effect today, but it has one drastic flaw: It pertains only to shelters in cities with a population of 10,000 or more. That leaves out much of Oklahoma.

When the mother-in-law learned of that law, she became nervous, and admitted that the adopters were planning on using Max for breeding purposes.

ON A HUNCH, Tammy checked out the back yard. Sure enough, in the middle of December, there sat Max outside, even though the "indoor only" box had been checked on the adoption application. Just one more lie, in a pile of lies, from people we—mistakenly—thought would be a good home. It has always been our policy not to adopt companion animals as outdoor pets.

Tammy went back to the shelter, where she summoned a police officer, who accompanied her, and Kennel Supervisor Bill Winchester, back to the home where the dog was reclaimed for breach of the adoption and sterilization contracts.

To his credit, Police Chief Robert Gillian, with whom I had had so many negative conversations concerning his poorly-run animal shelter, emphasized his determination to enforce the legislation.

"We'll take whatever action is appropriate to enforce state law," he told us.

Max was brought back safely to the shelter, where he and Jenny, another abandoned Boxer with only one eye, were adopted by Linda and her husband Dayman. Both dogs lived out the rest of their lives as members of a wonderful, caring home.

It turns out that if Max had been used for breeding, it most likely would have prematurely ended his life. It was discovered he had cardio myopathy, a serious heart condition, which may have been the catalyst that wound him up in an animal shelter in the first place.

Linda took Max to the specialists at OSU School of Veterinary Medicine, who advised her he would not live longer than a year, and he would be certain to have a sudden death.

The OSU veterinarians were right on one count. Max did suffer a sudden death. He had been outside in the yard with Linda, where he had not displayed any symptoms whatsoever, but when he came inside, right behind her, she heard a heavy thump.

"I knew what that sound was before I even turned around," she told me. Max was dead on the kitchen floor.

But the OSU veterinarians were wrong on the other count. Max had enjoyed eight years of a pampered life with his loving owners who faithfully administered his heart medication on a daily basis.

Try to imagine Max's life with that breeder who had lied on his adoption application. Would he have cared for a handicapped dog for all those years?

I don't think so!

In fact, if there was a top 10 list of reasons why Max was given up to an animal shelter in the first place, I wouldn't hesitate to guess that "unfit for breeding" was at the top of the list.

I tell this story for a number of reasons. First of all, Jenny and Max were both purebred Boxers. The AKC and breeders in this country want you to believe that purebred dogs and cats are not the problem. They don't end up in animal shelters.

Au contraire. Purebred dogs make up a surprisingly large percentage of animals that enter—and die—in animal shelters all over America.

Secondly, I think I can count on one hand the adoptions I have approved over the years that I am one hundred percent sure were good homes. It's not difficult to become cynical and distrustful of human beings when you lend yourself to the cause of animal welfare.

It is amazing, and disturbing, how often potential adopters lie on applications, just as they did in Max's case. Even though references they have provided can be checked, this is seldom good enough. And all too often, there are minimal background checks, or none at all, of the strangers standing before you, that you know absolutely nothing about, who say they are willing to take on the responsibility of the homeless dog or cat you have come to love.

I will say it again. I find it difficult to enter a PetSmart or other public facility where adoptions are underway, even though that's a good thing in many ways. There's nothing more rewarding than finding a good home for a homeless pet; but I fear too many of those dogs and cats will wind up in the wrong hands, just like Max almost did. Most humane organizations simply don't have the resources to complete thorough investigations of adoptive homes, and animals become losers for the second, third or fourth time.

I FOUND, IN one of my old plastic tubs, a police report dated July 8, 1987. After all the cruelties to animals I have witnessed in my thirty-five years of animal advocacy, I still found myself shocked at the report.

Cache, Oklahoma, is a very small community just west of Lawton. The humane society had received a complaint that a Cache city employee, who lived on the Cache landfill site, was taking cats from the local animal shelter and using them to train his coon hounds.

Our shelter personnel had also reported a man coming to the Lawton shelter, and inquiring if he could take animals from our shelter to his private landfill in Cache.

I reported this information to the chief of police in Cache.

The animal control officer of Cache was interviewed by the chief of police, who admitted that the man in question had, indeed, taken an undetermined number of cats, and two dogs, from his shelter. He said he was not sure of the amount, but stated, "they could not be counted on your fingers and toes."

The chief of police, accompanied by a deputy, visited the landfill to interview the man, who belligerently stated he had always used cats to train his coon hounds, but that he hadn't done it in a number of years.

The man then admitted he had taken two cats "a long time ago," but that he "still had them," although no cats could be located on his property.

When asked if he had ever gotten cats at the Lawton animal shelter, he denied ever going there for that purpose.

Cache animal shelter records revealed that the coon hunter had taken in excess of 20 cats from that shelter, in addition to others he had caught in traps in the yard of a friend.

Again, this is just one more instance of animals ending up in the wrong hands. These were unscreened cat adoptions, and these cats didn't die in animal shelters that euthanize.

If, however, anyone in the "no-kill" movement can tell me how mandatory neuter/spay laws, or humane euthanasia, is not superior to the deaths these cats suffered, while being killed by their adopter's coon-hunting hound dogs, I would be interested to hear it.

It will never be just about pet adoptions—or voluntary neutering and spaying. It has to be about laws that limit pet breeding!

This is America! We can do this!

CHAPTER 23

"An error does not become truth by reason of multiplied propagation, nor does truth become error because nobody sees it." — Mahatma Gandhi

THE NO-KILL MOVEMENT is an illusion which assuages the American conscience; and all too often, no-kill shelters pass out animals to just any takers, due to overcrowding of their facilities or a lack of "foster homes."

Even in 1997, Scott VanValkenburg, a young shelter worker from Seattle, realized this truth when he wrote a paper entitled "Towards A No-Kill Society: How No-Kill Shelter Declarations Hurt the Effort to end Companion Animal Overpopulation." It is a valid argument against the no-kill philosophy today.

"I killed my first dogs and cats eighteen years ago performing a merciful act that generates an intense emotional response that can only be completely understood by shelter workers," wrote VanValkenburg. "But it is long past time that sadness and anger crystallize to form a solution to the overpopulation of companion animals. Unfortunately, there is a growing chorus of criticism from within the animal protection movement directed at those who perform shelter euthanasia in this country. In the face of massive suffering and death of companion animals, it is time for aggressive campaigns. But the focus on so-called 'no-kill' declarations that are increasingly in vogue is actually hurting the effort to end the killing of ten million or more dogs and cats each year."

VanValkenburg chronicles the history of the need for humane animal shelters in America and condemns pet breeding, and the sale of dogs and cats as commodities. "As the humane movement grew, so did national campaigns to promote spay/neuter." he wrote. "With the development of the animal rights philosophy came more vigorous efforts to spay and neuter animals, and criticize breeding during the overpopulation crisis.

"The most important thing that those who want to end the killing of dogs and cats can do is vigorously campaign against the sale of dogs and cats, and to create a widespread consumer denigration of anyone who buys rather than adopts a companion animal."

He asserts that "no-kill" declarations interfere with the effort to focus the public on the immorality of treating dogs and cats as commodities . . . The effort to promote "no-kill" declarations focuses on symptoms of the crisis, and deflects public attention from the source.

VanValkenburg notes that the San Francisco SPCA, who are known for their stance on "no-kill" and have, to their credit, reduced the killing of animals in that city, fail to proclaim that they could have only taken the course they did because the city shelter continued to euthanize.

" . . . Just as ending the killing in one shelter building doesn't make a difference to the millions killed, neither does it make a difference if one city ends the killing without addressing the root causes of killing in their entire region," he wrote. "Teary-eyed donors divert money from spay/neuter programs to warehouses that hold a dozen or a hundred animals while thousands suffer and die around them. Dogs and cats are not meant to live in shelter situations, no matter how dedicated the individuals who work there or how wonderful the quarters. More importantly, sending money to care for a few individuals when the killing of millions can be ended is immoral."

After I read VanValkenburg's article, I was able to locate his phone number, and I called him at some point in 1998. We spoke on several occasions and could not have agreed more that adoptions are not, and never will be, the answer to the overpopulation problem. It's an important part of it, just not the end-all answer that the no kill movement wants us to believe it is.

IT'S THE BREEDING, stupid.

Those interested in politics may remember when Bill Clinton's campaign coined the phrase, "It's the economy, stupid," as a campaign slogan in his first run for President of The United States.

In the issue of an overpopulation of dogs and cats in America, it really is the breeding!

"Class, let's digest this slowly," said Professor John Goodfellow of the American National University of Pet Population Studies, in Gotebo, Oklahoma. "Research shows that dogs and cats multiply at many, many times the rate of humans. It is an indisputable fact that dogs and cats come into a heat cycle about twice a year, and have gestation periods of only two months. Sixty days!"

"Unlike humans, except perhaps for the infamous octomoms of the world," Dr. Goodfellow joked, attempting humor to spark a trace of interest in a half-asleep class of Animal Reproduction Studies students, "dogs and cats reproduce in litters. Often, alarmingly large litters."

"Now what have we learned here? Anyone? Anyone?" the professor asked, flailing his arms in frustration.

"Let's recap: Dogs and cats come in litters. Takes sixty days. Twice a year. Humans come, mostly, one at a time. Takes nine months," he said, as he paced around the classroom.

By now, the bespectacled academic was yelling—almost at the top of his voice—to a room full of would-be advocates for animal welfare. This was not Animal Reproduction Studies 101; these were students with years of undergraduate work in the subject matter of pet overpopulation.

"The science is solid. The math won't work. Too many dogs and cats," he shouted. "Not enough homes." Sadly, however, Dr. Goodfellow's students were uninterested in the truth.

Dr. Goodfellow ended his lecture in a calm, but defeated voice. "Even taking into account the fact that dogs and cats have shorter lives than humans, there is a principle of supply and demand here that is exceedingly unbalanced. Once again, class, the math just won't work!"

There is no American National University of Pet Population Studies. I made that up. To my knowledge, neither is there a Professor John Goodfellow.

There is, however, a Gotebo, Oklahoma, which is an insignificant dot on a map, and I would hope that students in Gotebo understand math and the law of supply and demand. When it concerns pet breeding and overpopulation, one plus one equals four, six, eight, or ten—with deadly consequences.

No matter how many celebrities get involved; or how much money is generated for animal care by tear-jerking TV commercials—who mention nothing about solutions; or how concentrated the efforts of the "no-kill" movement, reducing the pet population is the ultimate answer to the neglect, abuse, and killing of millions of pets in America. We can't adopt our way out of this.

No one is disputing the fact that we have had a pet overpopulation problem in this country for more than a hundred years. The problem is the lack of consensus among animal welfare advocates as to how we can end it. Adoptions and voluntary neutering and spaying—even high-volume, low-cost neutering and spaying—have been unable to stop the killing because we can't adopt, or neuter and spay, fast enough to overcome the ratio of dogs and cats to human beings.

Oklahoma ranks second in puppy mills in the nation. It's not uncommon for these facilities to house—in horrific conditions—more than five hundred breeding dogs. And that's just one state!

Without stopping the influx of millions of puppies and kittens onto the American landscape, we are just whistling Dixie. Nothing short of stiff, nationwide regulation of pet breeding, known as mandatory neuter/spay laws—with no exemptions or loopholes—will end the killing.

But getting these laws passed is tough business—considering the opposition.

The usual suspects who oppose laws to reduce the pet population—and thus the killing—are, of course, the purebred kennel and cat clubs; back-porch hobby breeders; and puppy mills.

Who might, however, not be expected to be found in the long list of opposing organizations are the American Veterinary Medical Association; breed rescues; and OMG, humane societies!

Yes, you read that right. Humane societies—lots and lots of humane societies—chief among them the ASPCA.

CHAPTER 24

"They're animals, all right. But why are you so goddam sure that makes us human beings?" — Stephen King, *The Long Walk*

"WE CAN'T DO this anymore," I said, sitting face to face with City Manager Melissa Vossmer. I had not made an appointment to see Ms. Vossmer. I had just shown up in her office, biting my tongue in an attempt to conceal my rage, over the fact that a dead baby calf had been left on the shelter grounds overnight.

OPERATING A MUNICIPAL animal shelter—or any kind of animal shelter—is perhaps one of the most stressful jobs on Planet Earth, especially if those who are running the shelter are there totally out of love and concern for animals—and not to extract a profit or simply to make a living.

You look at those beautiful dogs and cats placed in your care, who haven't committed any kind of sin, and who just want to go home, but you know full well most of them have no hope of home. All the future holds for them is death. That is a stressful job!

Add to that a war being waged against you by local veterinarians who didn't want you there in the first place—a war so bizarre as to almost be unbelievable; a war with veterinarians—are you ready for this?—over dead animals.

Yes. You read that right. Dead animals.

OUR CONTRACT WITH the City of Lawton specified that we provide appropriate containers "for the deposit of dead animals by any citizen or the City. All animals deposited in such containers shall be disposed of by Lessee in City's landfill site . . . Lessee shall not charge any fees for the deposit, collection, or disposal of such dead animals, and City will not charge lessee any landfill fees for such disposal. It is expressly understood by Lessee that the disposal of dead animals will be performed daily, and that no dead animals shall be placed or deposited into any of Lessee's solid waste containers, except in special containers provided herein."

The "appropriate containers" were, in fact, barrels that were placed on the shelter grounds for the use of citizens who needed to dispose of their dead dogs or cats. Most everyone has seen pictures of barrels, full of dead animals, in literature depicting the shame of pet overpopulation. It's not a pretty sight, but is an integral part of most shelter operations—adding, of course, another layer of emotional baggage to anyone who dares enter the world of animal welfare.

Historically, animal control had picked up animals that had been euthanized by veterinarians, and charged the veterinarians ten dollars at that time. (Today it is fifty dollars.) But it was a service provided by the city; and a fee was charged. We had no reason to think this would change.

Since we had taken over the shelter, the veterinarians—all except one—had, collectively, been depositing anywhere from a hundred to a hundred-and-fifty dead animals per week in the barrels. The manpower required to handle these dead animals, and the lime with which we were required to cover the bodies at the landfill, stretched our already inadequate budget.

The veterinarians argued that it was our duty to dispose of the dead animals they had euthanized in their practices, although our contract certainly was not explicit in the matter. It merely stated we would dispose of dead animals from "any citizen or the City."

One veterinarian, Dr. Roger Wyant, took the high road in the dead animal fiasco. Even though he had signed the petition that attempted to prevent us from taking over the shelter, he actually paid the humane society for the dead animal services.

"We just don't operate that way," he said. I remain grateful to this day for his courage to stand out from the crowd and defy his colleagues in this situation. The other veterinarians could have just as easily taken their dead animals to the landfill, as it was only a short distance from the shelter, but dumping them for us to handle, as a form of harassment, better fit their modus operandi.

"This is just not what we bargained for when we got into this," I said to Ms. Vossmer, choking back tears, as I was explaining about the dead baby calf, which, I felt sure, had been left at the shelter by a large animal veterinarian.

Ms. Vossmer did what she could to calm me in her office that morning. Although she was juggling political factions, she did what she could for us. In fact, at one time, in an attempt to help with our expenses, she personally provided the required lime with which to cover the dead animal bodies—or, at least, we were given that impression.

IN SPITE OF the veterinarians doing what they could to make our job difficult, it was amazing the support we were given by the community as a whole, and other communities in Oklahoma were seriously considering improving their animal sheltering duties, based on the example we had set.

A man from Ponca City, Oklahoma, wrote a letter to Ms. Vossmer, explaining he was on the board of his local humane society and chairman of the building committee.

"I am writing in reference to your new animal facility, which I recently saw on television. I am certainly impressed with what I saw," he wrote.

Ms. Vossmer responded to his letter by saying: "The improvements have been very much a joint project of the City of Lawton, the McMahon Foundation, and the Humane Society of Lawton-Comanche County." To say that it's a shame she was unable to add "local veterinarians" to that list is an understatement.

Four months into our operation of the shelter, we published *The Society News*, a small tabloid-sized newspaper. Pictured on the cover was longtime beloved Mayor Wayne Gilley with two small dogs in his lap, and five larger dogs at his feet. The caption read: "Mayor Gilley Loves Lawton, Its People, and Its Pets."

Today, as I look at those pictures of beautiful, gentle pets that we featured thoughout that paper, I can't help but wonder if we were able to get just even one of them a good home.

The cover story on the paper was entitled: "The Shelter Contract: Is It Working? We asked various city representatives, including the famed "Super Six,"as we had fondly dubbed six council members who had so strongly supported us, to express their views on whether or not they thought the contract was a good idea.

"I'm just all for it one hundred percent." Councilman Frank Walker beamed. "I'm looking forward to maybe someday tiling the kennels, and building a new cat kennel."

Councilman Bob Shanklin, who encouraged that Sunday demonstration, weighed in. "What I was interested in more than anything was the dedication of the people who were going to be involved . . . plus on paper it proves to cost us less money than for us to do it ourselves."

Councilman Keith Jackson said he thought that "the contract is working . . . and that since this was the first contract and it is working, we might explore other areas to contract."

Councilman Jeff Erwin gave us a glowing report. "I've never seen a more clean, more well-run and organized establishment. The people out there . . . are there to help. It used to be one of the most dismal, disorganized establishments that I have ever been in . . . Dismal, disorganized, and depressing. That's what it was. The three Ds."

Councilman Red Miller said he was "amazed at the change that has been made out there . . . I'm more than happy about what small part I had in it."

Councilman Gene Love: "It appears that everything is working out fine. I've not heard anything negative at all . . ."

Councilman Coleman Johnson was a bit reserved, but agreed that "at this point, I am pleased with the shelter contract and have had no reason for displeasure."

Even the three dissenting council members had nothing negative to say.

"From everything I hear, it seems the humane society is doing a great job," said Councilman Mel Fredricksen.

Councilwoman Leila Barfield said, "If it is working for the citizens, it is fine with me."

Councilman William Scearce said he had heard no complaints.

BUT IF WE were getting kudos from citizens, council members, and surrounding communities, we were getting nothing short of hell from Lawton veterinarians.

Dr. Joe Kiehn, one of our most vocal opponents, had even harassed us on fresh meat that was donated to feed the dogs. Martin's Steak House, the restaurant where we had entertained the Federal Trade Commission investigators from Dallas, had cleaned out their freezer and provided prime rib, steaks and other high end cuts of meat for the shelter dogs.

This came right before Thanksgiving, and I recall rising very early and cooking what seemed like a ton of meat for the dogs' Thanksgiving treat. A frozen food locker plant in Apache, a small town to the north of Lawton, also gave us a huge amount of ground beef.

Dr. Kiehn aired a complaint that this was not appropriate food for dogs—something to the effect that it wasn't a complete nutritional meal.

Well, golly! Dr. Kiehn must have forgotten this wasn't a lifetime diet for those dogs. Those dogs didn't have a lifetime. It was more like a last meal—before their execution!

CHAPTER 25

"You might want to think twice before you use a man's conscience against him. It may turn out he doesn't have one." — Brent Weeks, *American Fantasy Writer, The Black Prism*

WE TRIED TO take the veterinarians' criticism of just about everything we did in our stride. The hundreds of dead animals from veterinarians' practices, which were left at our gate, and in our dead animal barrels, was, however, too much to overlook; and the dead baby calf was the straw that broke the proverbial camel's back.

We had some tough decisions to make.

AROUND THE FIRST of July 1987, we met for a board meeting in which we discussed what we needed to do. We were running at least a two thousand dollar deficit every month and donations could not keep up with the needs. Council was not much interested in our request for a more fairly divided animal-related budget.

"We have been scraping and begging just to make payroll twice a month," Linda told the board. "Even though it makes us sick to think about losing the shelter and the humane care we know is given there, we cannot continue to operate at this deficit."

Linda pointed out that the entire budget for the department was $145,000, of which animal control received $100,000. Animal control at that time was manned by only two animal control officers and a dispatcher who worked out of the police department. On the other hand, over fifty percent of the animals that came into the shelter were never handled by the city, but were brought and left there by private citizens. We were performing the bulk of the tasks.

We had spent over $12,000 for capital improvements at the shelter, as well as receiving several thousand dollars-worth of appliances and supplies from supporters, and, if we left, this would all become property of the city.

"The sad part about all of this is that for the first time in many, many years this community has a good, humane animal shelter, and several other Oklahoma towns have called and visited our shelter as a good example," Linda told the board.

"But without some help very soon, this may all be lost. And, of course, as always, the greatest losers of all in these political battles are the animals themselves."

ON THE NIGHT before I would write the letter giving our thirty-day notice to discontinue operation of the city animal shelter, I paced for hours, in the moonlight, on the banks of the creek that surrounds my home, agonizing over the decision we had made.

I felt guilty. I felt I, personally, had let so many people down, including city council members that I had hounded to agree to this trial contract of city services; city staff; those people in other communities who had been so helpful and complimentary; and, of course, the supportive citizens who had given all they could in a city not known for its wealth. I felt I had betrayed all the beautiful pets that had come into the shelter, and the future ones who would have their time there, and die there, perhaps in a less humane manner than that which we had provided.

I felt I was a quitter.

My dear supportive husband allowed me to be alone for all that time on that warm summer night to sort things out. When I came into the house, however, he reminded me that the neuter/spay clinic was our best bet to help animals, and that we could somehow continue to operate the humane society along with the clinic. I knew he was right, but I got very little sleep that night.

On July 8, 1987, representing the humane society board, I wrote a letter to City Manager Vossmer, giving thirty-day notice of our decision to discontinue operation of the city animal shelter.

"Politics and power struggles have little or no place within the goals and purposes of a humane society, and the political issues and financial burdens involving the shelter operation have made it difficult, if not impossible, to keep sight of the higher goals and purposes of our organization," the letter stated.

Of course, the politics and power struggles of which I was writing came as a direct result of harassment from the veterinary community.

"The serious burden of dead animal disposal continues to remain unsolved," I wrote, "and we have repeatedly been unsuccessful in our requests for assistance . . . If the city chooses to continue this service, then so be it. The humane society, however, chooses not to."

We made it clear, however, in our letter that our decision by no means indicated that we had lost interest in the shelter and the welfare of the animals there.

We pointed out that relief from the financial and political burdens would better enable us to put a more concentrated effort on our neutering and spaying, humane education, and our goals of a anti-breeding, or litter law.

We sincerely thanked the council members who had been supportive, and acknowledged Ms. Vossmer's attempt to quiet the dead animal turmoil by paying for lime from her personal pocket.

BUT THE DEAD animal turmoil was not yet a dead issue.

On July 9, 1987, I submitted a requested op-ed piece for the Lawton newspaper for a point-counterpoint discussion of the situation.

The subject was: "Should Humane Societies or Others be Responsible for Veterinarians' Dead Animals? Below are excerpts from my article:

"Being aware of the strong opposition of Lawton veterinarians to the humane movement, it has been particularly vital for me to closely examine my feelings with regard to the question as to whether humane societies, taxpayers, cities, or anyone else should be required to haul off dead animals coming from veterinarians' clinics.

"I sincerely believe that if I were looking at the situation for the very first time today, and if I were not involved at all, I still would have to answer with an emphatic NO! Why should it be anyone else's job?

"This all, however, is now water under the bridge as far as the humane society is concerned.

We simply have said, 'we will no longer do it.' It's my guess that now that the city has the shelter back, veterinarians will at some point in the future be required to pay for this service, or will, on their own, take their animals to the landfill.

"There is little doubt in my mind that their insistence on dropping off the 100 to 150 dead animals per week at the shelter, for the past eight months, has been more to make our job difficult than anything else, considering the fact that they have been opposed to any humane movement that has ever been undertaken in this city.

"Lawton veterinarians have harassed veterinarians at the Animal Birth Control Clinic because of their opposition to a vital low-cost neuter/spay program, started by the Lawton United Volunteers for Animal Birth Control.

"We were not surprised, then, when Lawton veterinarians opposed an animal shelter run by the humane society. The dead animal disposal issue has been one of politics and harassment, more than contractual obligation, and it is a shame that 12 to 15 veterinarians can wreak so much havoc within a desperately needed humane cause . . ."

The op-ed piece ended with the following statement: "It's ironic that the Humane Society of Lawton-Comanche County and the Comanche County Veterinary Medical Association are battling over—God forgive us—dead animals!"

Dr. Wayne Haney, who, at that time was president of the Comanche County Veterinary Medical Association, presented his counterpoint. He argued that animal disposal was part of the contract operation requirement, neglecting to note that before the humane society operated the shelter, the city had charged the veterinarians to pick up and dispose of their dead animals—and continue to do so today.

"As a courtesy and without charge, the veterinarians have for years assisted residents in the proper disposal of a deceased pet," Haney wrote.

We doubted the validity of that claim because many people had told us they were charged. Others said they had been told by veterinarians their pets were being buried at a farm somewhere.

Dr. Haney expressed concern for citizens, or veterinarians, who might be required to transport a deceased pet to a landfill because of the chance of a "disease outbreak in the community, the spread of rabies, or any other disease the deceased animal might have."

He seemed to have no concern whatsoever for the health and safety of shelter workers, whose job it was to deal with those hundred to a hundred and fifty dead pets that he and other veterinarians insisted our shelter employees handle.

ON JULY 13, 1987, we sent out a newsletter to supporters in an attempt to explain our decision to bail out on the shelter.

"As I sit here on this rainy morning writing to you from the heart, I can't help but remember the beautiful animals that have crossed our lives during the past several months at the animal shelter. Many of the stories have happy endings like the injured, abandoned and abused animals that we were able to save and place in good homes. We have been criticized for our adoption policies, but could anyone fault us for attempting to make certain that we didn't put one of these innocent creatures back into a cruel situation for yet a second time?" I wrote.

"Our hearts break for those thousands of animals whose stories didn't end happily, and whose eternal destinies have been given up to God. For them, we did what we could, but our months at the shelter have brought home more than ever the tragic consequences of pet overpopulation.

"During the month of June, approximately 900 animals came into the shelter . . . old family pets not wanted any longer; tiny kittens and puppies, many with distemper and other diseases, that never should have been born in the first place.

Of these 900, nearly 800 were destined to end up at the city landfill, and for every animal put to sleep, a bit of us, whether shelter worker or humane society board member, died with it. It is a tragic shame that politics and greed can so greatly hamper a humane movement, when, if we all worked together we could accomplish so much for those who suffer the most—the animals.

"We will, however, put a renewed emphasis on our neuter/spay work because one day spent at the shelter would convince the most cynical skeptic about the desperate need for all pet owners to neuter and spay their pets. It is the answer to the killing. Please help us stop it by your support of our neuter/spay efforts, and supporting neuter/spay legislation and city ordinances."

IT SEEMED THE veterinarians had won this one. Their opposition, in the form of critical letters to council members, showing up at the shelter to take pictures, criticizing the occasional meat we fed the dogs, and flooding the shelter grounds with the bodies of dead dogs and cats—and baby calves—from their practices, had become too much for us.

Yes, they had won this battle, but would they win the war?

CHAPTER 26

"Think occasionally of the suffering of which you spare yourself the sight." — Albert Schweitzer

ALTHOUGH I WAS heartsick, thinking about the animals we would no longer be able to ensure would, at the minimum, have good meals and heartfelt hugs during their short stay with us, I was relieved that I was leaving that mass euthanasia behind.

Dan wouldn't talk to me about euthanasia. He would walk away if I attempted to bring up the subject. "I don't want to hear about it," he would say.

That is the reaction of most Americans to euthanasia of dogs and cats, however, we, as a nation, have done little to end the mass killing of millions of pets each year—over the course of a century.

Animal shelters, no matter who runs them, are not good places for animals. Whether it be a "no-kill" or a shelter that practices euthanasia, an animal shelter is not a home.

Even though we were doing everything in our power to make the city shelter a place of comforting love for the animals there, I still cringe when I think about the suffering of the animals. They came in with parvo and distemper. Uncaring animal control officers had no qualms about tossing a momma dog and her puppies on the searing hot metal of their caged-in pickup bed on a hundred-and-ten degree day in July. Some of the animals were afraid and sat quivering on the concrete floors in the chain-link kennels.

I will not forget, in this lifetime, one of a litter of tiny puppies that had fallen into one of the uncovered water drains inside the kennels. He had died in that drain during the night when no one was at the shelter. Who could ever have anticipated that cruelty? I had not seen the drains as any kind of danger. The architect who drew up the plans had obviously not viewed the drains as a threat to a shelter animal. These are things that most of us just never think about—and never want to know about—that happen every day in animal shelters throughout the country.

The answer is fewer animals, and thus fewer animal shelters—and, ultimately, less cruelty.

Of course, the clinic had been actively neutering and spaying while we were operating the animal shelter, but you can only stretch yourself so far; and we had neglected job one, which was to focus on solutions to the every day killing that was going on in our city—and which, for that matter, goes on day after day in every city and county throughout this nation.

After all, finding solutions to the killing was why we had organized that evening in 1984 in the first place.

What we had never anticipated was the tremendous opposition we were encountering from veterinarians on every front.

I asked myself again: "Just what is it that dead animals in a landfill bring to veterinarians' practices that they so desperately want to preserve?"

WE WERE SET to turn the shelter back over to the city the first week of August 1987. To say that we were bitter towards the veterinarians for their relentless battle against us—even at the animal shelter—is to put it mildly.

Their opposition to the neuter/spay clinic was, at least, understandable, but, in the name of God, what did they have to fear with regard to a humane society-operated animal shelter?

Oh, now I remember. It was just plain harassment! They would never forgive us for that clinic. Some of those who are still here haven't gotten over it to this day. And decades later, we would endure the wrath of the OSBVME in a manner we would never have even dreamed possible.

What they didn't understand was that being kept busy at the animal shelter actually put a damper on our attention to the neuter/spay work. It divided our emphasis.

Perhaps, too, what they didn't understand at the time was that, in a foolish attempt to try to get along with them, we had preliminarily declined to offer rabies vaccinations at the clinic. We did require the basic shots in order to protect all the animals that came into the clinic from the communicable diseases that could be prevented by vaccination; but early on we told customers they would have to go to a full-service clinic for their rabies vaccinations.

If the veterinarians had ever tried to sit down and talk to us, they might have found that we are fairly reasonable people; and our goal was never about hurting their business. It was about saving the lives of an overpopulation of dogs and cats.

However, now the practice of referring customers to other veterinarians for rabies vaccinations would no longer be the policy at the Animal Birth Control Clinic. It was off the table. We were taking off the gloves. We would sponsor a public vaccinations clinic—the day after we left the animal shelter—just to make a point. We would offer dog and cat vaccinations at a ridiculously low cost for anyone in the city, or surrounding communities.

Dr. Zdunek, our clinic doctor, along with assistants, agreed to administer the vaccinations; and my husband joyfully offered to purchase all the rabies vaccines. We would also use the car dealership as the location at which the event would be held.

So now we could advertise "Free Rabies Vaccinations for All Pets." The other basic set of vaccinations were offered for a mere five dollars.

The veterinarians wanted war? We were going to give it to them!

OF COURSE, THE veterinarians made sure that the health department came to the Animal Birth Control Clinic, before the day of the event, to inspect our vaccines and be sure they were from reputable pharmaceutical firms. They were. They still are today.

Oh, they have tried so hard, over the years, to find something . . . anything . . . oh, please, just anything, with which to snag us; and shut us down.

Two of them had shown up, with cameras, early one morning at the animal shelter to take pictures of the kennels. One side of the aisle had already been cleaned, but kennel workers had not yet gotten to the other side. Would you like to take a guess on which side of the row they took the pictures? You guessed it. The dirty side.

This was schoolboy nonsense, not the actions of full-grown professional men.

On April 29, 1993, after the Animal Birth Control Clinic had been successfully operating for eight years, Dr. Scott Briggs, wrote a letter to the Oklahoma State Board of Veterinary Medical Examiners, which he called a "formal complaint" against the clinic.

He stated: "My complaint is that the ABC Clinic is vaccinating pets owned by the general public and is charging for said vaccinations. Dr. Reynolds is only present at the ABC Clinic on Tuesdays and Thursdays of each week, yet pets are being vaccinated 5 days per week (Monday thru Friday) by unlicensed lay people who are signing Dr. Reynolds' name to the rabies certificate. This constitutes practicing Veterinary Medicine without a license and Dr. Reynolds is violating the Oklahoma Practice Act by permiting (sic) his name to be used in his abscense (sic).

"I request the Oklahoma Board of Veterinary Medical Examiners investigate this situation and take appropriate action the (sic) enforce the laws of the State of Oklahoma and the requirements of the Oklahoma Veterinary Practice Act as well as punish any guilty parties found." Obviously, Dr. Briggs' ages-old habit of telling people our doctors don't use anesthetic on surgery animals was not working. Time to try a new scheme.

The "illegal vaccination" trick didn't work either. Investigators from the OSBVME showed up at the clinic, with a subpoena, demanding our rabies books and vaccination records. They found nothing. Of course not. Honestly? Did they think we're stupid?

We have always realized we're under a magnifying glass, and one of the dumbest things we could ever do is have non-licensed persons administer vaccinations without a veterinarian present—or perform surgeries without anesthetic!

DAN ASKED EMPLOYEES to spit shine the dealership service department to get ready for the big event. We set up folding tables, on which we placed a small refrigerator filled with dog and cat vaccines, rabies books, and other record-keeping documents; we put large metal troughs into place with water hoses and bottles of flea and tick dip close by; and most of us donned scrub tops over our jeans. Then early that Saturday morning—just one day after we relinquished operation of the city animal shelter—the two large overhead doors of the service department were flung open to throngs of pet owners and their pets, who were lined up outside in the parking lot, and around the entire building, to take advantage of our offer of absolutely free rabies vaccinations—no strings attached!

"Oh my aching feet," Linda said, after a very long day of paperwork, and bathing and dipping countless numbers of dogs until almost dark. "I think I'm gonna have to crawl to my car."

That pretty much summed up the sentiments of all the volunteers and the doctor who worked so hard for animals in Lawton and Southwest Oklahoma that Saturday in August—thirty years ago.

We weren't done yet. We did the same thing again the next year at about the same time. This time our ads read: "Rabies vaccinations for only 99 cents." Dr. Reynolds was at the helm this year.

And, unashamedly, we held a low-cost rabies clinic the next year—for a third year in a row—wherein more than thirty volunteers helped vaccinate an excess of fourteen hundred dogs and cats.

We have offered complete sets of all vaccinations at the Animal Birth Control Clinic ever since; and I can't know this for sure, but I would guess we provide vaccinations to more dogs and cats than any other veterinary practice in Lawton and Southwest Oklahoma.

It's hard to feel guilty!

CHAPTER 27

"There's no guarantee that justice will win out or that a noble sacrifice will make any difference. But when it does, there's something that still swells my chest. There's magic in that...It tells me that's the way things are supposed to be." — Brent Weeks, *Beyond the Shadows*

FTC CHARGES OKLAHOMA STATE VETERINARY BOARD ILLEGALLY RESTRICTED COMPETITION: BOARD AGREES TO SETTLE CHARGES.

THAT WAS THE headline of the Federal Trade Commission press release of August 14, 1989. I remember the exact spot where I was standing in the clinic, early one morning, when Dr. Reynolds walked in and quietly handed me a DVM Magazine, its pages open to an article about an FTC ruling against Oklahoma veterinarians.

It's strange, but I don't remember jumping up and down; I don't remember gloating; I hadn't given much thought at all to the FTC over the past year or so. I remember being puzzled. What did this mean?

I picked up the phone and called the Dallas Regional Office of the Federal Trade Commission. I asked to speak to Ms. Malmberg, who agreed to fax me a copy of the press release.

There was a note from Ms. Malmberg on the cover sheet of the fax that read: "Mr. Kennedy will call you in about an hour to give you a chance to read this material."

As promised, in about an hour, I received a call from Gary Kennedy. I am not sure of his title. In my notes, I have written (title?) Mr. Kennedy explained that "the origin of the investigation is not public." That obviously meant they would not share with us what lead to their investigation of Oklahoma veterinarians as it pertained to the Animal Birth Control Clinic. We had always been under the impression it was sheer coincidence that they happened onto the clinic file at the Oklahoma State Board of Veterinary Medical Examiners, when they were performing routine investigations. We have no way of positively knowing, however, if that was the case. We will never be completely sure how they became involved. We only know the clinic was a big part of the investigation, if not the sole reason for it.

One thing is certain. I had nothing to do with the FTC involvement. To this day, I am accused by some of the veterinarians, who are still practicing here, of calling them. I would not even have known the FTC was the entity to investigate what was happening between Lawton veterinarians and the clinic.

Recently, when one of my dogs was being seen by my own veterinarian, we discussed, for a short time, the issue of pet overpopulation and the Animal Birth Control Clinic, and its colorful history.

My vet has a tremendous practice, and he is loved by his clients. For this reason, I think—I hope—he moved on quickly from his angst over the clinic—unlike most of the other vets that were here in those days. He conveyed to me that what veterinarians held against me—or still, to this day, hold against me, most of all, was the FTC investigation and ruling.

Well, yeah! That ruling pretty much changed the face of veterinarian medicine in Oklahoma. To use the language of former Vice-President Joe Biden, on one occasion, when he didn't know a nearby microphone was on: It's a "big fucking deal." It's what has allowed us to still be offering low-cost neuters and spays in Oklahoma thirty-five years later.

They had their nerve, however. They were caught red-handed violating the law, and they're still mad at me thirty-five years later?

Rather than writing out the Complaint and the Decision and Order, which are lengthy, the press release is condensed. It reads verbatim as follows:

"The Federal Trade Commission has charged the Oklahoma State Board of Veterinary Medical Examiners with injuring consumers by illegally restraining competition among veterinarians in the state. Under a consent agreement announced today for public comment, the Board agreed to settle the charges.

"The veterinary Board is the sole licensing authority for veterinarians in Oklahoma. The Board is a state government agency, but all of its members are full-time practicing veterinarians.

"The complaint charges that the Board restricted unreasonably the business arrangements under which veterinarians may practice. According to the complaint, the Board:

"—Prohibited veterinarians from forming partnerships with non-veterinarians if any of the partnership employment involved the practice of veterinary medicine; and

"—Prohibited veterinarians from accepting employment from a nonlicensed person, company or corporation which involved the sale of the veterinarian's services to the public.

"The complaint alleges that these rules hurt consumers by preventing veterinarians from offering more efficient business arrangements that could result in lower prices. The rules also hurt consumers by making it harder for qualified veterinarians to establish a practice.

"The complaint further charges that the Board unreasonably restricted the dissemination of certain truthful, nondeceptive information about veterinary products or services. The Board declared it to be unprofessional conduct for veterinarians to write testimonials about or endorse remedies, instruments, equipment or food, except to report the results of properly controlled experiments or studies for scientific journals or meetings, according to the complaint.

"The complaint charges that this restriction on disseminating truthful, nondeceptive information deprived consumers of the benefits such information can provide when consumers purchase veterinary products.

"Under the consent agreement, the Board agreed not to restrict veterinarians' business arrangements, but the Board may still prohibit interference by non-veterinarians with a veterinarian's professional judgment or integrity. The Board also agreed not to prohibit the displaying, offering, publishing, or advertising of any testimonials or endorsements by veterinarians with respect to any veterinary product or service.

"The Board is based in Oklahoma City. The FTC's Dallas Regional Office handled the investigations.

"The consent agreement is scheduled to appear in the Federal Register August 15. It will be subject to public comment for 60 days, until Oct. 16, after which the Commission will decide whether to make it final.

"Comments should be addressed to the Office of the Secretary, FTC, 6th St. and Pennsylvania Ave., N.W., Washington, D.C. 20580.

"A consent agreement is for settlement purposes only and does not constitute admission of a law violation. When the Commission issues a consent order on a final basis, it carries the force of law with respect to future actions. Each violation of such an order may result in a civil penalty of up to $10,000.

"Copies of the agreement, the complaint, and an analysis of the agreement are available from the FTC's Public Reference Branch, Room 130, 6th Street, and Pennsylvania Ave., N. W., Washington, D.C. 20580. 202-326-2222 TTY 202-326-2502."

MEDIA CONTACT: Susan Ticknor, Office of Public Affairs
202-326-2181
STAFF CONTACT Tom Carter, Dallas Regional Office
214-767-5503

Jim Elliott, Dallas Regional Office
214-767-5503
(FTC File No. 851-0047) (Okla Vets)

AND SO IT was that the Animal Birth Control Clinic, in the small Southwest community of Lawton, Oklahoma, could—in spite of unrelenting veterinarian opposition—continue to battle the tragedy of pet overpopulation by the only means available to them—by neutering and spaying as many dogs and cats as they could get their hands on.

That was a big fucking deal! That was divine intervention.

CHAPTER 28

"Veterinarians have had years to address this situation, and never have; and there are veterinarians in this state, associated with us right here, who make money by killing animals every week or month, or whatever they do. Then comes along people that have made their money legally and honestly, and they are doing their best to stop animal suffering, which is what we should be doing. And what do they get? They get slapped for it." — Dr. William Weber, Irondale, AL, during a hearing before the Alabama State Board of Veterinary Medical Examiners, regarding his work with the Alabama Spay/Neuter Clinic, July 2014

WITH REGARD TO veterinarians' fear and loathing of neuter/spay clinics, we thought our battle here in Oklahoma more than thirty years ago was as down and dirty as it gets; but it seems as if Alabama veterinarians make their Oklahoma counterparts look like choir boys.

The Federal Trade Commission ruling changed the manner in which the Oklahoma State Board of Veterinary Medical Examiners could place a stronghold on their members under their Rules of Professional Conduct—making it legal for a veterinarian to work for a non-licensed owner of a veterinary clinic, which, in our case, was a non-profit organization. That was 1989.

From our uneducated viewpoint, we were under the impression that that particular ruling had set a precedent, making it legal for low-cost neuter/spay clinics to operate across the country.

Unfortunately, that doesn't seem to be the case.

Alabama neuter/spay clinics were currently battling the exact same battle, under that state's practice act, with which we were faced in 1985.

An article in the July 2014 issue of *DVM360 Magazine*, bears the following headline: "Alabama state board finds veterinarian guilty after controversial hearing." The subtitle read: Charges in regard to Weber's supervision of Eastwood Animal Clinic became the center of the board's years-long public battle against nonprofit spay/neuter clinics."

The Alabama State Board of Veterinary Medical Examiners (ASBVME) had conducted a months-long administrative hearing and voted to revoke Dr.

Weber's license for a year, ordering him to pay a thousand-dollar fine for each of five guilty charges—for assisting Alabama Spay/Neuter Clinic in getting animals neutered and spayed.

"The administrative hearing began in January; the drawn-out process of interrogating Weber, run not by a third-party judge, but by the board itself, has caused some to term the hearings a "circus," the article stated.

Dr. Weber sat alone at a small table, facing his accusers, his arms folded in detectable defiance. After he had obviously had all the harassment he could take from his self-appointed prosecutors, the feisty, white-haired veterinarian valiantly defended his beliefs. Enunciating every syllable, he spoke in a loud, clear voice that often seemed breathless with frustration.

"You're taking minute details and minute dates, and trying to make mountains out of molehills," he told board members in the hearing, which can be seen on dvm360.com/weber.

"And the purpose is," he continued, "to try and squash the spay/neuter foundations, because, for some reason, you have it in your mind that the spay/neuter clinics, the low costs, are stealing money from veterinarians, which is absolutely hogwash," he said angrily.

"The great majority of these people," he said, referring to the people who use low-cost spay clinics, "are people that will never, ever go into a veterinarian clinic and pay five hundred dollars, or similar, to spay a cat that they are lucky they can feed, and catch in a trap and take it somewhere. They are not going to do that."

Dr. Weber praised spay/neuter clinics for "doing great good for homeless, stray animals that are dying in trailer parks, running all around restaurants, and getting killed under the dipsy dumpsters, and veterinarians have had years to address this situation, and never have."

The doctor, by now clearly outraged from days of endless grilling, pointed to one of the board members. "You get somebody like him, and some other people, that are just trying to take a magnifying glass and put it on every little word in the Practice Act, and calling it an infraction, and making me out a liar, a fraud, dishonest, and a whole bunch of other nice things.

"Veterinarians are not losing money from spay/neuter clinics. And if veterinarians would cooperate with them—cooperate," he emphasized in a firm loud voice, they would make money from them. "You be nice to some of these people, and they'll come back to you; and why people cannot see that is beyond me."

What have I been saying throughout this book? If the veterinarians would have just talked to us! But, alas, they have always preferred to fight.

"You can object 'til your glasses fall off, but you're not going to shut me up," continued the good doctor during his rant, amid numerous objections from the attorney for the board.

"How can a veterinarian go to school and learn surgery, and come out with no compassion?" he asked in an increasingly agitated voice. "There are veterinarians in this state who have a hole in their brains where compassion ought to be, and they are trying to fill it up with money."

One of the attorneys for the board asked Dr. Weber if he believed any of this "excuses you from the law."

In a raised voice, Dr. Weber answered emphatically, "I DO NOT."

THE BATTLE IN Alabama has raged for years. A September 13, 2013, article, written by Julie Scheidegger, in *DVM360 Magazine* is entitled "President of the Alabama state board sues VMA: Battle continues to wage on in veterinary community."

Alabama veterinarians are not only fighting low-cost neuter/spay clinics in their state; it seems they are waging war against each other.

"The relentless battle of nonprofit spay-neuter clinics in Alabama continues on the pages of lawsuits and subpoenas," Scheidegger begins. The article states that the president of the ASBVME, Robert Pitman, DVM, sued the Alabama Veterinary Medical Association (ALVMA) in June, stating that the association engaged in "conduct not in the interest of members."

Dr. Pitman, under a contract with the City of Athens, is the operator of the Athens Dog Pound, where he is paid for sheltering—and euthanizing—stray dogs and cats.

According to the DVM360 article, this fight had been fought in the Alabama Legislature, but left both sides without a victory, when the legislative session ended without passage of either a Senate bill backed by the ASBVME, or a House Bill backed by the ALVMA. Legislators said they couldn't get a feel for what the majority of veterinarians wanted.

Ms. Scheidegger points out that the veterinarians had taken sides with the ASBVME and the allied Alabama Veterinary Practice Owners Association (AVPOA) who both desire a very limited role for nonprofit clinics—some believing there is no place for them at all—or with the ALVMA, which wants to establish defined but fair regulations for the state's four clinics that meet appropriate standards of care.

"Technically, it's still illegal for the Alabama Spay/Neuter Clinic to operate with a 'nonveterinary' owner," said ALVMA president Bill Allen.

SEVERAL MONTHS AGO, when I first learned of the veterinarian harassment of the neuter/spay clinics in Alabama, I was mesmerized at how similar—but even uglier—the Alabama case was to our battle with veterinarians here in Oklahoma thirty years ago. If I had even entertained a thought that, in all these years, the veterinarians' position on neuter/spay clinics had evolved, or they, as a professional community, had become even infinitesimally enlightened with regard to the societal ills of pet overpopulation to both animals and humans, I obviously was foolishly mistaken.

I called and spoke to the director of the Alabama Neuter/Spay Clinic, one of four low-cost clinics in that state, and offered him all the information I had on the FTC ruling in Oklahoma. He seemed excited to receive the material, and conveyed to me that he would pass it on to their attorney. I faxed the information that same morning, but I heard nothing more from him.

After I read of Dr. Weber's controversial hearing before the ASBVME, and watched the internet video, I placed a call to Chris Waller, Dr. Weber's attorney. Waller, who seemed to have a genuine passion for the plight of his client, and the cause of the neuter/spay clinics, informed me that another attorney for the Alabama Spay/Neuter Clinic had contacted the FTC, and was working with them in an attempt to get a resolution to the controversial rules of the Alabama Veterinary Practice Act.

OVER THE YEARS, Dr. Reynolds has kept me abreast of articles in the *DVM360 Magazine* that seem pertinent to the neuter/spay cause. The latest article is from the September 2014, issue, entitled:

"Ala. Spay/neuter vet appointed to ASBVME: In an ironic twist, Dr. Margaret Ferrell, a target of the Alabama state board, is appointed by the Governor to serve on it." This piece was also written by Julie Scheidegger.

"It's safe to say that virtually everyone with a stake in the highly publicized, political and controversial debate on the role of low-cost spay/neuter clinics in Alabama was, at the very least, surprised when Gov. Robert Bentley appointed the newest members of the Alabama State Board of Veterinary Medical Examiners (ASBVME). Even the most notable appointee herself, Margaret Ferrell, DVM, says she did not expect the call," wrote Scheidegger.

What? The Governor of Alabama appointed the very veterinarian who works for Dr. Weber, performing neuters and spays at the Alabama Spay/Neuter Clinic, and who is, herself, charged with a thirty-three page administrative complaint by the ASBVME for her work at the clinic?

Could there be some divine intervention at work in the State of Alabama?

The appointment, according to Scheidegger, came on the heels of Dr. Weber's hearing, which he has appealed to the Fifteenth Judicial Circuit Court in Montgomery.

According to the article, Governor Bentley's office put out a statement that Ferrell "is well qualified and brings a wealth of experience to the board. Obviously, he was aware of the complaint, but chose to move forward. He has a good deal of respect for her."

In a quirky twist of fate, Dr. Ferrell will take the place of Dr. Robert Pitman, who is the outgoing president of the ASBVME, and, from all indications, the most notorious leader of the push against low-cost neuter/spay clinics—at least in Alabama. Unfortunately, veterinarians with the mind-set of Dr. Pitman are all over the place!

According to the Limestone County Animal Control website, Dr. Pitman has contracted, since November 1, 2003, with Limestone County to operate the Athens Dog Pound (yes, it is referred to as a dog pound) to "receive, house and dispose of animals delivered to him by animal control."

Now wouldn't you just think that someone—anyone—who has been operating a shelter/killing house since 2003—especially a veterinarian—might by now see the need for high-volume, low-cost neuter/spay clinics. Would he not be weary of the killing?

It didn't take me that long to figure it out. What's wrong with Dr. Pitman?

In September 2011, The Huntsville Times printed an article by writer Keith Clines, which states that Dr. Pitman had asked the Limestone County Commission and the City of Athens for $287,860 to continue the services at the Athens Dog Pound. The article said Dr. Pitman had originally asked for $400,000, but revised his request.

I keep asking over and over again: What is it that dead animals bring to veterinarians' practices that they have fought so hard, for so long, to protect? Perhaps I've just found the answer, at least in the case of Dr. Robert Pitman, veterinarian from Alabama.

Dr. Weber, one of those veterinarians who gets it, was right on in his description of the kangaroo court in which he was tried by the ASBVME in Alabama.

Animals are dying, by the millions, day after day, year after year, all across America—in the midst of this nonsensical "hogwash."

CHAPTER 29

"It's not about going around trying to stir up trouble. As long as you're honest and you articulate what you believe to be true, somebody, somewhere, will become your enemy whether you like it or not."
— Criss Jami, Rock Singer, Author, *Venus in Arms*

IN JULY 1987, the city council voted to advertise for bids for a new operator for the animal shelter.

City Manager Vossmer also announced that the city had hired Randall Riggs, a young man from Winfield, Kansas, as assistant city manager.

Three of the ten council members voted against advertising for bids, saying they preferred a staff recommendation that the city resume control of the facility.

Ultimately, council voted to advertise for bids, along with the city staff recommendation to include a budget of $63,830. The city staff also recommended an oversight committee composed of members of the humane society, veterinarians, city staff and the city at large; and giving shelter control to the assistant city manager.

Council discussed the ongoing dead animal issue.

"Why should the city provide this service for private business?" Councilman Frank Walker asked, referring to the veterinarians using the shelter "as a dumping ground for their dead animals." The council voted, however, to continue the service of taxpayers shouldering the bill for disposal of veterinarians' dead animals.

The city contracted with the Lawton Animal League, a newly-formed for-profit organization. To put it mildly, our feelings were hurt—no, actually, we were miffed—when we learned that the city had agreed to pay the for-profit people considerably more than the amount with which we had been operating.

While it is true that the city was in a crippling budget crunch at the time they originally agreed to contract with us, we had told them ahead of time we would be unable to renew at the current deficit. City staff had made it clear, however, that we could not and should not expect more money in a renewed contract.

We would not have minded the increase for the Lawton Animal League if it had meant the animals would benefit. But that was a pipe dream. Animals benefitting from a for-profit organization?

I don't think so!

NO SOONER WAS the ink dry on their contract, when the Lawton Animal League started making statements, via the media, that they, unlike the humane society, would not be creating controversy. Like a host of angels, swooping down across the city, with harps playing strains of the "Hallelujah Chorus," they would get along with everyone—to include veterinarians, city staff, and especially newly hired Assistant City Manager Randy Riggs, with whom, it would turn out, they would have an unusually cozy relationship.

While it was true that since we stepped into the picture at the city animal shelter, it had, indeed, been the subject of much-heated controversy, and had evoked more emotion than perhaps any other area of municipal government. Considering the ages-old killing of thousands of innocent dogs and cats, it was as if we had awakened a collective conscience within the city.

But, as we found out when we established the low-cost neuter/spay clinic, and then set out to raise the awareness of the failings at the city shelter, not everyone is going to be on your side.

Controversy was not something we were chasing, but we weren't running away from it either.

I was angered by an article in the newspaper wherein a staff member of the Lawton Animal League again criticized the humane society, inferring that we were at odds not only with city staff, but the world in general.

"Let's set the record straight." I said in a letter to the editor. "The controversy was not created by the humane society, but by a private interest group which erroneously believes that any effort for animals is an infringement on their private businesses. In any instance, where private business and animals are concerned, you can bet the animals will take a back seat to monetary consideration. "It has never been our desire to intentionally create controversy, but we have refused to succumb to the pressures of private interest, thus creating controversy. For these same reasons of remaining independent, effective and uncompromising in our principles, we declined to serve on the recently-appointed shelter advisory committee.

"It's true that change never comes easily or without pain. The controversy of the past, however, has brought the animal shelter to the attention of those who need it most—city officials. It also has brought to this community high quality, low-cost neuter/spay surgery, which is vital to solving the single most tragic animal problem today—pet overpopulation.

"If the controversy surrounding the humane society has served to change even in a small way the deplorable conditions that have existed for animals in this community for years, then let the controversy continue.

"The Humane Society of Lawton-Comanche County will unashamedly be at the center of it!"

Soon enough, however, the Lawton Animal League would find themselves embroiled knee deep in their own controversy—and it wasn't for any of the right reasons.

IT WAS NOT difficult to understand how the Lawton Animal League was able to get along with the veterinarians. They were actually being financially backed by them—or at least one of them.

Months into the contract, when the Lawton Animal League was being scrutinized for their financial accounting—or lack thereof—they admitted to members of the oversight committee that Dr. Woesner had loaned them the initial capital with which to obtain the shelter contract.

Dr. Woesner? The veterinarian who sat on the original committee assigned to study the feasibility of contracting out the shelter to our organization? The one who said all stray dogs and cats are criminals, and the "majority need to be euthanaized" with an emphasis on the word "need?"

That same Dr. Woesner now had a financial interest in the Lawton Animal Shelter?

He had been doggedly opposed to contracting out the shelter to a non-profit humane society; but now he was backing a for-profit group—for more money? Where was that concern for Lawton taxpayers, which he had so righteously vocalized only a year or so earlier?

THE HUMANE SOCIETY received a letter dated August 31, 1987, just one month after we had relinquished operation of the city shelter, from Asssistant City Manager Riggs, stating that we had outstanding debts to eight veterinarians for vaccination certificates of adopted shelter animals.

After a thorough checking of her records, Linda sent a reply to Riggs, indicating payment in full to all veterinarians. "The Humane Society has always been and will always be good for our debts." she wrote. "If the veterinarians claim to have any further outstanding coupons, they must furnish us names, dates, amounts and services to allow us to check back into our records."

It became quickly obvious it was a good idea to check the veterinarians' billing. Linda noted in her response, dates and check numbers where coupons had been paid. She had deducted sixteen dollars from one veterinarian's invoice because his dog had been impounded by animal control, and he had refused to pay the humane society the impound fee, simply walking out with the dog.

She also noted that Dr. Woesner had submitted a twenty-five-dollar spay coupon for which no spay had been performed. "We checked with the owner of the cat that had died under his care, but we paid the twenty-five to the owner as the coupon was not meant to be used for any services other than a neuter or spay," she noted next to the billing. She enclosed a copy of the coupon.

City Manager Vossmer neglected to pay for the lime she had volunteered. We absorbed that bill.

We were never billed again by the veterinarians; and another stray had died at Dr. Woesner's clinic.

CHAPTER 30

"Follow the path of the unsafe, independent thinker. Expose your ideas to the dangers of controversy. Speak your mind and fear less the label of 'crackpot' than the stigma of conformity. And on issues that seem important to you, stand up and be counted at any cost." — Chauncey Depew, American politician, 1834-1928

IN NOVEMBER 1988, Dan and I purchased *The Lawton Times*, a small, weekly newspaper. Okay. I admit it. It had occurred to me that owning a newspaper would be a great bully pulpit for a cause—say perhaps the cause of animal welfare.

Besides, the veterinarians were circling the wagons. Dr. Joe Kiehn had secured for himself a seat on the city council, and, rather than recusing himself, was taking the lead in animal issues.

Dr. Dan Woesner of "all strays are criminals and need to be euthanized" fame had financially backed the for-profit Lawton Animal League. Dr. Wayne Haney was serving as the Animal Advisory Committee chairman. He had also written the counterpoint op-ed piece on why taxpayers should pay to dispose of veterinarians' dead animals; and he later threatened Sharon Methvin, vice-chair of the committee, for questioning the finances of the Lawton Animal League. These were veterinarians who had not been friends of our humane movement in Lawton.

The Lawton Times had been around for years. Its owners, Matt and Marcy Haag, had planned to discontinue publishing the paper, as they were reaping little financial rewards for their labors.

Our offer to buy *The Lawton Times* came with the stipulation that Matt and Marcy stay on and work for us. I had published a local monthly magazine about ten years prior to that time, but knew little about newspaper layout and publishing. We needed their years of experience and skills.

We put together a talented staff. Freelancers—both writers and artists— came out of the woodwork to be a part of this endeavor. We were members of the Oklahoma Press Association and The National Newspaper Association. We wrote about local politics, people profiles, and human interest stories. Perhaps my proudest contribution to the paper was an interview I was able to get with Larry Jones, founder of the International Charity, Feed the Children, headquartered in Oklahoma City—a man I greatly admired.

We carried well-known nationally syndicated columnists such as Andy Rooney and Lars-Erik Nelson, as well as columns by The Oklahoma Observer editor and publisher, Frosty Troy.

We were a small, but viable, newspaper and, in the words of Fox News, fair and balanced. As an example, we gave space to local veterinarian, Dr. Don Beavers, on the occasion of his being named president of the Oklahoma Veterinary Medical Board during its seventy-fifth annual convention in Stillwater; and when the police chief, with whom we had fought so many battles, did something right, perhaps in the local war on drugs, he received credit in an editorial.

But, yes, we published the hell out of animal issues. The daily newspaper had given us precious little support, and we worried that the covert antics of veterinarians-turned-politicians would never ever see the light of day. We had learned a few things in the daily chaotic atmosphere in which we had been forced to function.

If you wore a name tag that read press, you could ask questions of government officials. Of course, any citizen should be allowed to ask the same questions, but those people don't pose as much of a threat to bureaucrats, and others, as those who buy ink by the barrel, as the saying goes. Being a small newspaper, our printing was "jobbed" out, but we were still buying ink.

I don't think *The Lawton Times* ever turned a profit. The publishing business is a tough one, especially in a small community. We were, however, able to squeak by, which was good enough for me—because I had a larger agenda. As usual, my husband was a hundred percent supportive.

IF YOU TRY to please everyone, you please no one. I learned that years ago.

I remember Sharon Methvin, an instructor at the local college, as a petite, quiet-spoken woman, who truly cared about the humane treatment of animals. She had been one of the initiators of the Animal Advisory Committee and served as its vice-chair.

"Deloris," Sharon had told me proudly. "I'm going to get along with everyone." Oh, Joy to the World! Everyone is going to get along.

"That's great, Sharon," I forced myself to say in an upbeat tone. "Yeah, good luck with that," my brain was silently thinking.

A few months into her service as vice-chair on the advisory committee, Sharon was finding that getting along with everyone was not proving to be as easy as she perhaps had thought. In fact, sticking her neck out on the committee would later result in her need to hire an attorney to represent her.

Sharon may have started out naive, but she was an intelligent woman, and she was not liking what she was observing, both on the committee and at the shelter.

She insisted that Assistant City Manager Randy Riggs, who was charged with monitoring shelter operations and contract compliance, had turned a deaf ear to any complaints from members of the committee; and that the committee itself was laced with conflicts of interest. She accused the committee of protecting the profits of those it was intended to monitor.

"I have been asking Randy Riggs for a complete accounting of the Lawton Animal League's finances for well over a year now," Sharon told *The Lawton Times*, in an indepth article we printed on the controversy.

We asked Keith Aycock, a local attorney, and member of the humane society board at the time, and now a district judge, to attend a committee meeting when Sharon, and one or two other committee members, had become frustrated with chairman Haney and Riggs.

Aycock said that after being asked to attend his first meeting, he got very interested in what was going on and started attending meetings on his own.

"The thing that concerned me," Aycock said, "was that I would ask Mr. Riggs if monthly financial reports had been made as specifically required by the contract and he would tell me they hadn't."

According to Aycock, a request had been made of council to change the contract wherein the monthly reporting would become a quarterly reporting. He said the council was told the Lawton Animal League was in compliance with all reporting requests.

"The Lawton Animal League was not in compliance," Aycock said. "And when the subject came up in the spring about the audit, the city staff opposed the audit.

"I was initially led to believe that monthly financial reports did exist and I sent a letter in September 1988, asking for the reports," he said. "The reports were never furnished, and that is when I finally attended another meeting and asked Mr. Riggs, face to face, if any reports had ever been furnished, and was told they didn't exist."

According to Aycock, the performance bond had been waived, without consent of council, because the Lawton Animal League had been unable to obtain either a performance bond or a letter of credit.

"The performance bond was then deleted from the present contract." he said. "Here now all this money is short and yet it was city staff that recommended the performance bond be stricken from the contract.

"It was a cover up from the beginning and they are now trying to put the blame on someone else."

Aycock said his interest in the animal shelter situation was heightened when Methvin obtained his services to defend a complaint made against her by Councilman Joe Kiehn, on behalf of the Lawton Animal League.

"I was contacted by Sharon to obtain a copy of the complaint and was advised that no formal complaint had been filed," Aycock said. "I think the timing of it was interesting because Sharon was the one who made the motion to have the Lawton Animal League provide the audit, and she pushed hard for it.

"It was right after that that this complaint was allegedly made. It's my understanding that she was advised by Chairman Haney of the complaint and she could either have a hearing or resign. I think they dropped it after they found she had obtained an attorney."

Dr. Haney also had problems with members of the humane society, as well as attorney Aycock, showing up at committee meetings—even though they were open to the public. At the end of the meetings, audience participation was permitted and we always had questions. Dr. Haney was overheard telling a couple of committee members that something had to be done about limiting audience participation.

"I've tried to shut her up before but couldn't do it," committee member John Gossett of VAPS had chimed into that conversation.

"It would be nice if someone in this town could shut her up," Haney had said.

Who were they talking about? Was it me? Was it Vickie Warren, an outspoken animal advocate, who had attended most meetings as an observer and a vocal participant? It couldn't have been Sharon Methvin as she was on the committee.

It was probably me.

ON MARCH 28, 1989, the city council voted to give the Lawton Animal League 90-day notice that their contract would not be renewed. Assistant City Manager Riggs described it as two years of "continuing controversy."

Controversy? Oh, I thought we were all going to get along.

At a May 23, 1989, Lawton City Council meeting, nine council members, including Councilman Joe Kiehn, DVM., voted to raise the state-mandated animal shelter adoption deposit back to thirty-five dollars, up from the required minimum deposit of ten dollars, which was charged by the Lawton Animal League.

A ten-dollar deposit was not an incentive for adopters to comply with the state law that shelter animals be neutered and spayed, but it increased the amount shelter operators could place in their for-profit pockets on adoptions. Sharon Methvin and the humane society had opposed the ten-dollar deposit.

Not only did Councilman Kiehn vote to raise the deposit, but he suggested that the city now charge veterinarians for picking up their dead animals and taking them to the landfill.

Whoa! When the humane society was no longer at the shelter, Dr. Kiehn was now advocating veterinarians to pay the city for removal of their dead animals—just as it had been in the past!

THE CITY TOOK back control of the animal shelter July 1, 1989. The 1989-90 budget for animal control increased again. That same budget called for the termination of twenty city employees.

Who would ever connect the elimination of twenty jobs within a municipality to the problem of pet overpopulation? There is a distinct connection.

The dark, ugly tentacles of pet breeding, whether accidental or intentional, reach deep and unsuspected into society in ways few can—or will—permit themselves to even comprehend.

CHAPTER 31

"Throughout history, it has been the inaction of those who could have acted; the indifference of those who should have known better; the silence of the voice of justice when it mattered most; that has made it possible for evil to triumph." — Haile Selassie, Emperor of Ethiopia

THE FINANCIAL RECORDS of the Lawton Animal League had concerned us; but we had bigger fish on our plate at that time. Sharon was having to fight that battle by herself, along with Attorney Aycock, who proved to be a tremendous help—to both the humane society and the Animal Birth Control Clinic.

On July 6, 1987, at about the same time we gave our 30-day notice to the city that we would not renew our contract, the humane society received a call regarding six greyhound dogs, belonging to a City of Lawton employee.

Helen Tedder, the rainy night phantom of milk crates and wooden pallets, and I met officers at the location, which had previously been a meat butchering plant.

The police report accurately described what we saw: "A pen with six large greyhound dogs in it. The pen was very nasty with trash and a small amount of food, and very little water. The water that was there was sour and solid green in color. There was also a large amount of flies present. At request of Delores (sic) Delluomo animal control was called to pick up dogs. Also picked up was one pit bull dog. Officers located the dogs' owner and issued him a summons."

So far. So good. We had been able to get the dogs out of that unholy mess in which they had been condemned to barely exist.

When we received the dogs at the shelter, we immediately went to work caring for those poor, abused animals. Clean food and water was what they needed most, but they needed veterinary care, to include deworming and vaccinations. Probably, for the first time in their lives, those pitiful creatures had soft blankets on which to lay their tired, aching, prominently protruding bones.

A court date had been set for Mr. A. O. "Dodie" Cooper, owner of the dogs, in Municipal Court. Before that date, however, the humane society had already left the shelter, but the dogs were still there—and in great shape by that time.

Knowing that we were watching the activities at the animal shelter, and with cruelty charges pending, we felt the greyhounds would be properly cared for in our absence.

But, as we've learned over the years, when it comes to trusting people with animals, never take anything for granted.

No sooner had the humane society exited the shelter, animal control officers, who admitted to being friends with the owner, released the dogs back to him—while cruelty charges were still pending—and in violation of several city codes.

Cooper was ultimately found guilty of animal cruelty and ordered to pay a two-hundred-dollar fine—a mere slap on the wrist. Thanks to animal control officers, the dogs were back in the hands of their abuser.

Almost exactly one year later, in July of 1988, the humane society received yet another call that dogs in this same location were "starving to death." Once again, we found these same dogs, along with five others, for a total of eleven emaciated animals.

And, once again, police removed the dogs and placed them back in the city shelter—this time under the care of the Lawton Animal League.

We were pushing hard for this repeat offender to be prosecuted to the full extent of the law, this time pressuring the district attorney to take the case to district court. We were, however, getting the run around from everyone involved.

A veterinarian report by Dr. Haney, and Dr. Sam Moore, another local veterinarian, who had also been a thorn in the side of the Animal Birth Control Clinic, was the reason given by District Attorney Robert Schulte and City Prosecutor Sue Taylor for no cruelty charges being filed.

The police department had refused to let the humane society view their report from Drs. Haney and Moore, but what they didn't know is that an employee at the shelter had shared with us what was in the report—and we also had our own veterinarian report.

We had asked Dr. Reynolds, who was working at Southwest Veterinary Clinic in Elgin on his days off from the clinic, to go to the shelter and examine the eleven dogs on July 8, 1988. Dr. Reynolds submitted an in-depth report of his observations at the Lawton Animal Shelter.

On August 22, 1988, I wrote a letter to District Attorney Schulte, on behalf of the eleven dogs. "As per our recent conversation regarding the A. O. Cooper case involving malnourished dogs, enclosed is Dr. Kenneth Reynolds' report as you requested."

"As you will notice, Dr. Reynolds stated the condition of each animal as he found it. Unlike Dr. Wayne Haney and Dr. Sam Moore, who were hired by the city, Dr. Reynolds refrained from making judgment calls as to whether the man in question is merely "ignorant" or possibly "cruel."

I told the district attorney that Drs. Haney and Moore had determined that Cooper was not so much guilty of animal cruelty as he was "ignorant."

The two doctors' report indicated there were wounds on one of the dogs that they attributed to fighting. The report states that the wounds had healed due to the "excellent care" of their owner.

"I am extremely hard pressed to understand how Drs. Haney and Moore could state the dogs had received 'excellent care' for wounds and in the same report attribute their findings of emaciation, dehydration, flea and tick infestation and temperature elevation to 'ignorance' of the owner. It would seem Drs. Haney and Moore would realize that one who is competent enough to afford good care in treating wounds would be competent enough to simply provide adequate food, water and shelter—especially when a judge advised him of that necessity a year earlier," I wrote.

"Mr. Schulte, as I indicated to you on the phone, there are too many questionable areas in this matter for it to be dropped. You are aware, of course, that the man in question is a city employee and was shown favoritism last year when his animals were returned to him in violation of several city codes and while cruelty charges were pending against him—charges that later resulted in his being found guilty of animal cruelty in municipal court.

"I spoke a week or so ago to Mr. Randy Riggs, assistant city manager, who advised me no city employees have even been reprimanded for their illegal actions in this case.

"We are, of course, distraught that city hall is taking such a light view of this breaking of the law by city employees, i.e. animal control personnel, and believe that the police department, because of their blunders, is relieved that no charges of cruelty are to be brought against Mr. Cooper by your office.

"We believe that in view of the extremely contradictory report by the veterinarians hired by the city (Dr. Haney incidentally is with a clinic used by the city for veterinarian work for years, and I understand he was allowed to choose the second veterinarian, both of whom we believe to not be unbiased in their analysis of this matter,) available photographs taken of the dogs at the time they were confiscated, a number of credible witnesses, the fact that the same individual was found guilty of cruelty in 1987 involving several of the same dogs, and the additional report by Dr. Kenneth Reynolds of Southwest Veterinary Clinic, that your office should again review the case and reconsider your decision not to prosecute.

"The animals in question are now dead and nothing can alleviate the hunger and suffering these animals most likely endured, much of it caused by their illegal return to their owner by city employees, who openly claim to be friends of Mr. Cooper. "However, actions taken today may eliminate the further suffering of other animals.

"Again, I implore you," I wrote, "in the name of those who have no voice in the matter and in light of evidence set forth above, please reconsider bringing charges of animal cruelty against Mr. Cooper."

I included an afterthought, in the form of a P.S. at the bottom of the letter: "As I mentioned to you on the phone, video footage by Channel 7 is also available of these dogs and the conditions in which they were confined. Also, may I remind you that the dogs were removed from the premises by the police department at the initial investigation, action that in itself indicates the dire conditions of the animals at the time."

Copies of the letter went to City Manager Vossmer; Assistant City Manager Riggs; all city council members; the Lawton Constitution/Morning Press; KSWO TV; PETA and the Animal Legal Defense Fund, both in Washington, DC—and the Animal Advisory Committee.

WHEN IT WAS obvious there was not going to be any prosecution of this man, I contacted PETA to see if there was something they could do. Below are excerpts of the August 11, 1988, letter written by a PETA representative to District Attorney Schulte:

"People for the Ethical Treatment of Animals (PETA), the nation's largest animal rights organization with over 250,000 members would like to request that charges of animal cruelty be brought against Mr. Dodie Cooper for the alleged abuse he has inflicted upon the 11 dogs that were confiscated approximately one month ago.

"We understand that these eleven dogs were involved in an animal cruelty case against (the dog's owner) in 1987. In this case, (the dog's owner) was found guilty of animal cruelty and ordered to pay a $200 fine. These same eleven dogs, when confiscated approximately one month ago, were found to be emaciated, dehydrated, and had open sores on their bodies. Mrs. Dolores (sic) Delluomo, President of the Humane Society of Lawton/Comanche County, informs us that credible witnesses, a veterinarian's report, photographs and videotape are all available to document these allegations of animal cruelty.

"We are pleased that the dogs are now in the custody of the police department, and that Mr. Cooper is being charged with operating a kennel without a permit, and failure to properly vaccinate his animals, however due to the seriousness of this abuse we respectfully request that animal cruelty charges be brought against Mr. Cooper. Anything less would not do justice for the years of suffering that these eleven dogs have endured."

The letter was signed by Kyle Owens, an investigator for PETA, with copies to Sue Taylor, the city prosecutor and to me, as president of the humane society.

Owens also made a call to Police Chief Gillian, after the chief had advised me by phone that they intended, once again, to return the dogs to their owner after he paid his fines.

Shortly, after that call, Mr. Cooper released the dogs to The Lawton Animal League and they were euthanized within the hour.

That same day, I also sent a lengthy memo to Animal Advisory Committee members. I told them, according to veterinarian reports, the dogs were again infested with worms, but never dewormed during the eleven-day stay at the shelter. I shared with them that I was "appalled by this fact, considering the monetary profits being enjoyed by shelter operators."

I wrote in the memo that "I was surprised and saddened to learn, through Sharon Methvin, that the Animal Advisory Committee had not even been made aware of this situation, especially when those at the scene included the assistant city manager, a city council member, three police units, two animal control units, three humane society members, and a photographer hired by the humane society; and that the veterinarian hired by the city to examine the dogs is chairman of the Animal Advisory Committee."

I attached a computer printout of animal control citations from January 1, 1988, through August 16, 1988, indicating only two (2) citations were issued during that time for cruelty in the entire City of Lawton.

"The humane society receives at least three calls a week," I told the committee, "and our experience reveals that not only should citations be issued, but in many cases offenders should be in jail."

Animal cruelty in the City of Lawton was not or never had been a priority of the Lawton Police Department, Lawton Animal Control, the local district attorney, or even the then-chairman of the Animal Advisory Committee, Dr. Haney—a veterinarian. It still isn't today.

Sadly, the same can be said of thousands of communities throughout the United States.

CHAPTER 32

"To me, cruelty is the worst of human sins. Once we accept that a living creature has feelings and suffers pain, then by knowingly and deliberately inflicting suffering on that creature, we are guilty, whether it be human or animal." — Jane Goodall

THE GREYHOUND CASE was only one of dozens of cruelty cases that were all but ignored by animal control in Lawton.

With the memo sent to committee members about the greyhounds, I included a copy of a statement from Lawton woman, Sharon Hegna, that I had received just a month before. The statement is self-explanatory:

"On July 29, 1988, I Sharon Hegna called the police department around 7:00 or 7:30 p.m. to report a dog that was down and appeared to be sick. The dispatcher put me on hold for about a minute, then came back on the line and I told her there was a dog in the yard behind us that was sick and I thought the dog might be covered in ticks and didn't know wheather (sic) he would make it through the night. She replied ma'am there is not anyone on duty after 5:00 p.m. that could come out. Again, I stated that the dog wouldn't move and there wasn't anyone at the house where the dog was. The dispatcher again said there is no one that could come out and if there was they couldn't go in the yard and do anything without the owner being there. I would have to call back on Saturday. Morning at 8:00 a.m.

"While I was talking to the dispatcher, she started talking to someone else . . . The phone call to the police was made from our neighbors house . . . I had gone over to their house trying to find someone that could help. They made some calls trying to get some information. I then called Deloris Delluomo and she immediately came over and took the dog to the vet. By the time she arrived at the vets' office the dog died."

This pitiful, weakened dog did indeed die in the back seat of my car before I could get it to a veterinarian.

My next stop was to the police department to make sure they saw this dead dog whose body was completely covered in ticks—the dying animal that did not merit an animal control response!

Never once was I asked where the animal was found, in order to cite the owner, and as far as I know, he never paid a penalty for what he had allowed that dog to suffer. The two officers were more interested in making excuses for not responding to the call than in gathering information about the owner.

"Do you agree that citations for animal neglect and other violations of city codes are as important as traffic citations?" I asked committee members in the memo.

"Setting aside animal suffering, citations issued for animal violations are also means of revenue for the city and I believe that the taxpayers deserve them to be enforced," I wrote.

"Ladies and gentlemen of the committee, our animal related problems are massive. I invite you to answer the phones at the humane society for only one day, and, I believe, you would be convinced that we must address these problems for the sake of the community, the taxpayers, and the animals."

Just five months later, in February, we checked out a call where we found a sheltie mix who was very thin, pregnant, extremely weak and chained beside a dog house. The weather was brutal, with heavy winds dropping the chill factor into the single digits.

The dog belonged to a man who, we learned, was in the military. We attempted to talk to the owner of the dog, but he was loud and verbally abusive, using four-letter words to me and another volunteer. He went into his house and produced a bag of cheap dog food, to indicate the dog was not starving, which he proceeded to throw at me.

We pointed out the weak condition of the dog, and its need for veterinary care and warmth, and he grabbed the poor little animal and literally stuffed it into the dog house. He told us he couldn't afford veterinary care and that "the damn dog is going to die anyway. It has parvo."

We called the police department who came and gave the humane society authority to take the animal to a veterinarian for help, but before help could be reached the animal died in my car.

This was the second dog to die in my car in the past six months.

I asked Dr. Reynolds to perform an autopsy, which indicated that the dog was suffering from enteritis, an inflammation in the wall of the intestinal tract, and also from peritonitis, which is an inflammation or infection of the lining of the wall of the abdomen. The dog was also dehydrated.

Perhaps this man became worried about being in trouble. He called the humane society later that evening and explained to a volunteer that he has always handled animals in that manner, and that back where he was from, they just "let pets die to weed them out."

On April 3, 1989, I wrote a letter to a Captain Carmen, the soldier's company commander at Fort Sill, in which I explained the man's inhumane behavior towards this dog. "We do feel you should be advised of his behavior to humane society volunteers, but more importantly, we are most concerned about his attitude to helpless animals.

"We would hope that (this soldier) would give considerable thought before bringing another pet into a situation where it cannot be properly cared for and where pets are allowed to be "weeded out" in this manner," I wrote.

I can't say whether this animal abuser ever had charges brought against him; or whether his company commander even addressed the issue with him. My guess would be: No!

THE FUNDAMENTAL QUESTION that comes to mind when I see dogs or cats mistreated in this manner is: How did they wind up in those kinds of homes? Were these dogs animal shelter adoptions? Did they come from a weekend adopt-a-thon? Were they "free to good home" dogs?

Linda and I, as well as a few others in our organization, including most of our employees, have always taken the stand that we prefer humane euthanasia to taking a chance on placing animals in questionable homes—homes where they were forced to endure an unfulfilled need for simple food, clean water, warmth, and human love and companionship. That is the life of horrific suffering and death the above dogs endured.

That revelation always gets us flack from the no-kill community. It just, simply, is the truth. One of our policies regarding euthanasia at the animal shelter—and today at the clinic—is that an animal that came in starved or abused should be given a longer period of time to ensure it some positive quality of life. An animal being euthanized should be waging its tail in response to being surrounded by the love of those who have been caring for it, and who are performing the euthanasia.

Until we stop the overproduction of animals in this nation, that, sadly, is the best we can do. Yes, we have been criticized for our strict adoption policies.

As for me, I stand firmly behind them. Animal shelters are full of adoptions gone bad!

CHAPTER 33

"At first, they'll only dislike what you say, but the more correct you start sounding, the more they'll dislike you." — Chris Jami

I WAS SAD to learn, from the Internet, that Jan Vickers had died in 1998, only nine years after she had served as supervisor of Lawton's animal shelter. When I knew her twenty-four years ago, she was a likable woman, with a subtle sense of humor and a mischievous grin, and she knew how to work her way around the good old boy system. She was smart and well-educated, with a master's degree in psychology from Pepperdine University.

I think it was Sharon Methvin that got wind that Vickers might possibly be interested in coming to Lawton. Sharon was working hard on getting the city to hire an experienced, humane supervisor for the animal shelter.

On April 10, 1989, she sent a letter to Assistant City Manager Riggs advising him she had attended a conference with a number of humane educators and animal control officers; and that she would be happy to furnish him publications that could be used to advertise for a qualified shelter director.

Jan had worked for both the Albuquerque, New Mexico Animal Humane Association, and for the City of Albuquerque, in the development of animal welfare programs.

The City of Lawton hired her on July 3, 1989, as supervisor of animal sheltering—after the exit of the Lawton Animal League. Animal control services remained under the supervision of the Lawton Police Department.

On August 25, that same year, City Manager Vossmer resigned her position to take an assistant city manager position for the City of Waco. Before she left, she had set the wheels in motion to make Vickers supervisor of animal control—to give Jan the whole ball of wax.

Bob Bigham, who was acting interim city manager for the time between the Lawton Animal League and the hiring of Vickers, was on board with the decision, as were city attorneys. Bigham said the shift would mean better treatment for the animals.

Vickers would be taking on considerably more responsibility with no increase in pay, saving taxpayers money.

But the usual whiners went to work. Dr. Joe Kiehn, veterinarian, said the decision should be a council decision. He said he had heard rumors that the "lady" at the animal shelter didn't care for some of the animal control officers, and he feared for their jobs should she become their supervisor. I think Vickers, indeed, would have had problems with momma dogs and puppies on hot metal pickup truck beds on a 110-degree summer day in Oklahoma.

Police Chief Robert Gillian was also dead set against the move. Animal control was a thorn in the side of the police department, but, somehow, they didn't want to give up the pain.

I had a file full of complaints from citizens about animal control officers' treatment of animals.

The Cooper greyhound case, and the dog, dying in its own back yard from ticks, was only the tip of the iceberg.

These were the type of incidents that had endeared me (not) to animal control and the police department for years. If I knew about it, I was going to make a stink about it. I was sick and tired of getting calls, as a volunteer, and doing the jobs of others who were being paid. A few years down the road I would pay dearly for my years of speaking out. Not once, but twice.

IN SPITE OF all the evidence to the contrary, Dr. Kiehn said animal control was doing a "good job" and should be left alone—the same message he had disseminated three years earlier when the humane society wanted to operate the then-deplorable animal shelter.

Insiders knew, however, that Councilman Kiehn's greatest fear was that Vickers would be too chummy with the humane society, as she had made it known that she intended to work with animal welfare organizations, a decision that anyone who cares about animals should respect.

Jan and I did become friends. She visited in our home, and became friends with my family. Together, we went out on freezing, cold, nights on complaints of cruelty due to lack of proper shelter, a job she often took on voluntarily without asking for overtime. This was in addition to her duties at the shelter, and while animal control officers were snuggled warm in their beds and paid overtime when they went out after 5:00 p.m.

Of course, Jan cared about animals. That was the basic difference.

Jan was able to get almost every bite of food, fed to the animals at the shelter, donated—a feat that not only saved tax dollars, but allowed a pet on death row to have a good meal. She was responsible for the installation of donated water coolers for the summer; and she managed to get the city to purchase a professional animal control vehicle, which was enclosed, with air-conditioned and heated kennels.

Jan admitted that animal issues are not going to go away. "We have to deal with it, and deal with it now. That, unfortunately, has to be done through city and state politics."

She had plans to bring out-of-state experts to Lawton, such as Dr. Alice DeGroot, a retired Albuquerque veterinarian. Dr. DeGroot traveled nationwide at the time as a consultant to humane societies and shelters. She was a friend of Jan's so there would be no charge to the city.

She also planned to bring to Lawton Phyllis Wright, Vice-President of Companion Animals with the Humane Society of the United States, with whom she shared a friendship. She also was an acquaintance with Ingrid Newkirk of PETA.

Wow! Had we scored a big one or what? I, and others, including, I believe, city staff were thrilled that Jan had agreed to come to Lawton. She was a catch.

OF COURSE, NOT everyone shared our enthusiasm about our new animal shelter supervisor. Dr. Joe Kiehn and his buddies were successful in preventing animal control from being transferred to Jan's jurisdiction—even though she was a certified animal control officer.

He was relentless in his opposition to just about anything she attempted to do at the animal shelter. Although he kept a relatively low profile during regular council sessions, he obviously practiced his politics best behind the scenes. He threw up roadblocks in any issue aimed at reducing the killing at the animal shelter.

Jan had made arrangements, with one of KSWO TV 7's reporters, to produce a documentary film to be used as an educational tool depicting the inner workings of the shelter, to include the everyday process of euthanasia.

She had also enlisted the consultation services of her friend, Phyllis Wright, of HSUS. This was a coup for the city, not only because Wright had a more-than-hectic schedule, and was in ill health, but, also, because she was not charging the city for her services, thanks to Jan.

The filming was not a sinister plot, nor a secret to be kept from council members or city staff. It was, merely, being produced as an educational tool and part of a package to be presented to council members at a workshop planned during Wright's visit to Lawton.

On the day before the filming, however, Vickers was told by Interim City Manager Bob Bigham that her project was being postponed—apparently mostly due to the objection of Councilman Joe Kiehn.

This was also Dr. Joe Kiehn, veterinarian. He extolled the virtues of often less-than-humane animal control officers, and was vocal in support of the Lawton Animal League, whose operation of the city shelter was laced with contractual violations and questionable financial audits.

CHAPTER 34

"And the fox said to the little prince: men have forgotten this truth, but you must not forget it. You become responsible, forever, for what you have tamed." — Antoine de Saint-Exupery, French writer and poet, *The Little Prince*

"I WAS STANDING in front of the deep metal sink filled with surgical instruments and syringes that had accumulated in a massive heap, thanks to procrastination. I hadn't worked at the veterinary clinic long, and I was still getting the feel of things. The smell inside the surgery room was a unique one. A combination of Uritrol, used as a disinfectant in mop water, and the sour, sharp smell of vitamin B complex and other medicines, inhibited a chemically clean odor that made my nose hairs tingle.

"As I vigorously scrubbed at dried blood on a pair of forceps, my eyes browsed over different bottles of medication on the shelves above the sink. A bright red label caught my attention. It read "Sleep-A-Way." Below this name was a white skull and crossbones with the word 'POISON' printed on each side.

"I put the sudsy, clean forceps on the rinse side and picked up a pair of iodine-stained towel clamps. I thought they must use this drug to put old, weary dogs out of their misery. What an appropriate name.

"Eventually, I began to move up the steps in succession to assume more responsibility, the same pay, and unfortunately, more nasty chores. One of which was taking out the trash. This may seem like an ordinarily simple task, but at a veterinary clinic, you never know what will turn up.

"One day I came to work after school, as usual, and Dr. (name withheld), my boss, told me to dispose of a bag on the surgery table. I went into the room and picked up a heavy, black trash bag. This bag was so compact and dense that I found it difficult to carry. The bumpy contents were warm against my body and this overwhelmed me with a bizarre feeling. Trash that was body temperature.

"Before long I had received the dubious honor of seeing what went into these bags: a dog, a cat, some old and thin, some young and playful. I tried not to let my feelings get to me. I imagined it as simply work and something that had to be done. Occasionally, this concentration would be broken by the bad aim of the doctor who lowered the dead animal into the thin plastic casket I held. A paw might miss the intended target and brush limply against my arm. As I repeatedly saw these helpless, dead animals going into the bags, I realized the extent of lives being wasted.

"Pet owners would bring in animals to be put to sleep, some with justifiable reasons. Maybe Spot was 97 in doggie years and was growing so old and feeble that it was a struggle for him to go to his bowl. Unfortunately, most cases were not so easily acceptable. A pet would be in excellent health, but was considered a nuisance. This nuisance was disposed of in the most convenient manner—kill it. These instances were difficult on the entire veterinary staff. We would keep the younger pets and try to give them away to caring families. While each pet waited for a happy, new home, everyone would become attached to the cute, little puppy or kitty. Time would eventually take its toll and if a home didn't present itself, Dr. (name withheld) had no other alternative but to kill our new little, unsuspecting friend.

"I will never forget my last day of work at the clinic. I was rushing around finishing up for the day, when a dirty, two-tone blue Chevy pickup truck pulled around the back. It came to a stop and a little blonde, country girl eased out of the passenger door. Her long hair needed attention and her soft, round face was flushed from crying. I walked with her in silence to the back of the truck, where she pointed at a cage. Inside it was nine light-colored kittens and two long-haired Persian mother cats. The mothers watched contently (sic) over their onery (sic) but cute babies. Blam! The back door slammed and the girl and I turned to see Dr. (name withheld) and her mother walking towards us. He nodded to the older woman and pointed in the back of the truck in question. She nodded back to confirm the cats were in the cage. Together, the doctor and I lifted the cage out and set it on the ground. The little girl looked back hesitantly, then climbed into the truck and they drove away. Dr. (name withheld) looked at me reluctantly. He slowly withdrew the bottle of 'Sleep-A-Way' from his overalls pocket. Neither of us said a word, we both knew what the other was thinking, 'we have no other choice,' and we did our job.

"If the pet owner would only assume more responsibility to have their pet 'fixed,' unwanted animals wouldn't be produced. By planning ahead, they could eliminate extensive fees, humane guilt and the trauma involved with letting an animal sleep-a-way. In the eloquent words of Bob Barker of 'The Price is Right,' Please have your pet spayed or neutered."

Those old plastic containers in my closet give up so much history. I have no clue as to why I have the above written words of a freshmen student at Oklahoma State University in one of those tubs.

It is dated October 9, 1991, and was obviously an English essay assignment. The name of the student is right at the top of the paper, however, I will not reveal it because I have no idea what his circumstances are today. Whoever he is today, he was an insightful young man in his college days. It was his choice to withhold the name of the veterinarian.

Pet overpopulation has traumatized so many for so long. In this case, it is the young freshmen college student, the tearful child and her mother, and the veterinarian who took the responsibility to perform the painful, disgraceful job; or it is something as insidious as the twenty city employees who lost their jobs due to budget crunches even though the budget for animal control was increased.

That was 1991. Fast forward to 2020. The dates are of no significance. In spite of the ofttimes futile efforts of tens of thousands engaged in the battle against pet overpopulation, pick-up trucks still pull up to the doors of humane societies, animal shelters, veterinarians—and off to the side of an isolated, county road— and leave behind the tragic consequences of unregulated pet breeding.

This is America. We can do better than this!

CHAPTER 35

"Compassion is not religious business, it is human business, it is
not luxury, it is essential for our own peace and mental stability, it is
essential for human survival. — Dalai Lama

IN JANUARY 1990, Robert Hopkins was hired as Lawton's new city manager.
I liked him a lot. If he wasn't a bleeding heart for animals, he at least understood
what we were trying to do; and, I think he respected it. If this was to be his city,
why would he not want every department to be as efficient as possible.

Jan also got along great with Hopkins. They both had that quirky sense of
humor. Although he was unable to get animal control under her supervision, he
recognized there was a problem; and, in time, he would fix it.

There was no way, however, we were going to be able to keep someone of
Jan Vicker's caliber and expertise in Lawton, especially with the politics and
veterinarian harassment she was experiencing. To get the door slammed by Dr.
Joe Kiehn, on something as credible—and benign—as teaming up with the local
television station to make a much-needed documentary of the inner workings of
a local animal shelter, along with getting a big shot from the Humane Society
of the United States to help her, was not only mean-spirited; it was downright
immoral.

But what else was new in Lawton America—at least in the field of animal
welfare?

Jan toughed it out for about eighteen months and went back to Albuquerque
to take a job with the Bernalillo County Animal Control.

On April 15, 1991, Patti Hilliard from Wichita Falls, Texas, was hired by the
City of Lawton as its next animal welfare supervisor. Notice the upgrade in the
name of the division: Animal Welfare. Maybe we were making progress after all.

Patti was a protégé of Toni DeStephano and the Wichita Falls Humane
Society. She had her head screwed on right when it came to good animal welfare
policies, and we all had confidence in her with regard to animal sheltering. From
the beginning, however, I worried that she might not be assertive enough to take
the harassment she would undoubtedly receive from the old brigade—the good

old boys—in light of the fact that she would be taking over the supervision of the animal control officers.

Yes. Finally. Animal control would no longer be under the supervision of the police department.

That was a good day for the animals of Lawton, Oklahoma.

City Manager Bob Hopkins was making much-needed changes to the hierarchy of the Animal Welfare Division.

A very kind letter to the Humane Society, addressed to my attention, dated April 17, 1991, from Bill Baker, Public Works Director, outlined the city manager's plans.

"As you are aware," Mr. Baker wrote, "Ms. Patti Hilliard was hired by the City of Lawton as Animal Welfare Supervisor on April 15, 1991. The City plans to combine the Animal Shelter and Animal Control activities under Ms. Hilliard's supervision in the very near future. The City Manager's proposed reorganization, places the Animal Welfare Division under my operational/management control as Environmental Services Director."

"I have asked Patti to contact you within the next several days to discuss goals and objectives of the animal welfare issue in our community. It is my intent to cooperate fully with your organization and others sharing the same concerns. We encourage your assistance and request your suggestions. We want to work with you for the benefit of the animals and, of course, the citizens.

"I would like to ask one other thing. If, at anytime, you or members of your organization think that we are doing something wrong, or, if you have ideas or suggestions, please call Patti, or me.

"I assure you that we will thoroughly investigate any problem, carefully evaluate any suggestion, and respond to you in a timely manner.

"Thank you for your interest, concern, and dedication to the animals."

The last sentence of Baker's letter were words we had been longing to hear from Lawton veterinarians for the past six years: "Working together I know we can make great progress."

Again, a letter to the Humane Society of Lawton-Comanche County, was addressed to my attention and dated September 17, 1991, from Public Works Director Baker. Except for dates and names, this letter and the one dated five months earlier on April 17, 1991, were almost identical. This time, however, Mr. Baker had scratched through "Ms. Delluomo," in the salutation and handwritten "Dear Deloris." I was getting a good feel about Bill Baker. I think the city was trying to work with us. Looking back to those days, I think maybe they always did try. It was veterinarians who threw the kinks in the works.

This letter began: "As you know, Mr. Jerry Owens was hired by the City of Lawton as Animal Welfare Supervisor on September 17, 1991. In accordance with the recent reorganization, the Animal Control and Animal Welfare Divisions were consolidated under my operational/management control as Environmental Services Director. Mr. Owens will be directly responsible for supervision of the division."

Once more, the letter ended with: "Working together I know we can make great progress." Just as I had suspected, Patti, with all her love for animals and experience in animal sheltering, had been no match for the police-department-trained animal control officers.

The City of Lawton was going through animal shelter supervisors as fast as the Animal Birth Control Clinic had gone through veterinarians before the Federal Trade Commission ruling, but there was no doubt they were trying to get it right.

Today, as I look back at how cooperative most city officials were to us back then and compare it to what happened here in 2015, twenty-four years after Baker's letters were written, it is astonishing. City officials, rather than admit the city's negligence in a tax-supported animal shelter once again riddled with unspeakable inhumanities, allowed a corrupt OSBVME investigator, burdened with glaring conflicts of interest, to frame concerned citizens for fabricated crimes while protecting animal shelter supervisors and others he was enlisted to investigate.

CHAPTER 36

"Very little of the great cruelty shown by men can really be attributed to cruel instinct. Most of it comes from thoughtlessness or inherited habit. The roots of cruelty, therefore, are not so much strong as widespread. But the time must come when inhumanity protected by custom and thoughtlessness will succumb before humanity championed by thought. Let us work that this time may come. — Albert Schweitzer

IT SOMETIMES GIVES me a headache to revisit the information contained in my plastic tubs. More to the point, it gives me a heartache. It seems that everything—everything!—we have tried to do was steeped in controversy. It's a verified fact that change doesn't come without pain, but does it have to come with so much pain?

In 1990, five of the ten Lawton City Council members voted for a "no-chain" ordinance. Council members Frank Walker, Keith Jackson, Leila Barfield, Ron Nance and Alvis Kennedy all voted to ban chaining. Dr. Joe Kiehn, veterinarian, Minnette Page, Jerry Shelton, E. R. Kirby, and Jim Branscum voted to allow pet owners to continue to chain their dogs. It was a tie.

This law was heavily-fought—evidenced by the fact that only half of the council members voted in favor of it. That was the lowest percentage rate we'd had on issues we had presented to city hall.

We couldn't find many such laws in the entire United States on which to base a no-chain law. To get it passed was a major feat that didn't come easy. We had talked to Jeff Wilkinson, a young animal control officer, who had been able to convince his city leaders into a similar law for the small community of Maumelle, Arkansas, but other such laws were hard—if not impossible—to find.

On June 12, 1990, Mayor Bob Shanklin, who the humane society had strongly supported, and *The Lawton Times* had endorsed in his campaign for mayor, broke the council tie, and voted in favor of the anti-chaining proposal. This is what we would have expected from the former councilman who recommended we picket the city shelter in 1986.

By the next morning, on a Wednesday, he was threatening to veto the ordinance, stating he had not been prepared to break the tie. The following Friday he assured several of us he would not exercise his power of the veto, however, the following Tuesday he did just that. He vetoed the ordinance—a first in Lawton's history.

Never before in Lawton's freakin' history—since its beginning in 1901!—had a mayor ever vetoed a council action. What the hell was going on?

There had to be more at play here than met the surface. It was about this time that we had started rumblings about licensing and "litter" ordinances that would start to regulate pet breeding in Lawton. Almost two years later, in April, 1992, council would pass the law, but, in spite of an intensive campaign, we would never see it enforced. It's incredible how politics played into everything we tried to do. Pet breeding had rarely ever been challenged—just as it is rarely challenged today. We didn't get into this cause, however, to preserve the status quo.

One of the four reasons, listed by Shanklin, for vetoing the ordinance was that an advertisement had been placed in the local media criticizing council members who had voted against the ordinance. He said the ad was vindictive. It was an ad we had placed; and I was surprised that he was surprised. We always fought hard—but fair—for animal-related causes. He knew that.

Councilman Walker said we've got a problem when we euthanize 10,000 animals a year. He said the veto was totally uncalled for and that it was a definite action to keep the mayor's "clique together."

Shanklin's "clique" would have been the Dr. Joe Kiehn faction. I can't say why. Again, it's politics. It could have been a quid pro quo sort of deal. Perhaps because the clique agreed with Shanklin on other issues, such as capital improvement projects and wastewater treatment plant issues, he had to go along with the Joe Kiehn anti-anything-animal group.

Veteran Councilman Jackson said "any time a public figure starts reacting to paid advertisements in the media by vetoing council action, you've got to wonder who he represents."

Councilman Alvis Kennedy said he felt sorry for animals "who have to sit out in this heat on chains. We owed it to the animals to get them off chains."

Linda, as a spokesperson for the humane society, was quoted in the newspaper: "What was his motivation in vetoing his own vote? Whose interests are really being served by this veto? One thing is for sure. He has done the pit bull fighters of Lawton a definite service."

Linda said she took offense to the mayor's citing of a humane society advertisement as one of his reasons for vetoing the ordinance. "The humane society has always, when we can afford it, made a habit of publicizing individual council member's decisions on animal issues. It was a positive ad meant to give credit where credit was due—and otherwise.

"When someone goes into office, they risk criticism," Linda said. "I believe we call that Democracy."

The daily newspaper editorialized on the issue of a no-chain law. Retired Lawton Constitution editor Ted Ralston wrote an op-ed piece about stopping "The Pet Brouhaha at City Hall." Ralston said the ordinance "represents an overreaction that has been typical of animal rights activists here for some time."

Oh, an overreaction of animal activists; not veterinarians?

I took on Mr. Ralston with my own editorial in *The Lawton Times*. Is it becoming clear why I wanted to purchase this newspaper?

"One can only guess that Mr. Ralston rarely sees a dog on a chain in his fashionable west side neighborhood," I wrote. "And we can be almost certain that Lawton's pit bull breeders who produce fighting stock (albeit a felony in this state) never keep their dogs on heavy tractor chains (as is the practice of many pit bull owners) anywhere near Mr. Ralston's home.

"And it is possible, but highly improbable," I continued, "that Mr. Ralston has heard about the Goodyear employee who applauded Mayor Shanklin's veto last week, and then bragged this week to fellow workers that he had left town for the week-end, (just about the time we were reading Mr. Ralston's comments) and returned to find his chained dog dead in the heat.

"And we can't help but wonder whether Mr. Ralston ever in his life answered a call in sub-zero weather to a tiny alley apartment on C Avenue to find a weakened, pregnant and seriously ill Sheltie chained to an inadequate doghouse. Would Mr. Ralston's view of the chaining law be softened if this Sheltie had died in the seat of his automobile because he couldn't get her medical attention fast enough?

"And, of course, Mr. Ralston couldn't know about the dog chained to the clothesline pole on Euclid last summer, who died from the heat and lack of water—on the same afternoon that an animal control officer had been there and done nothing. Or, about the female pit bull, found only days later, chained on West Lee. She was saved, but only after her male counterpart had died—another animal control blunder."

I wrote that these are not isolated incidents. "They happen so frequently, Mr. Ralston, that sometimes it gets to be more than those of us who 'overreact' can stomach."

I pointed out that Mr. Ralston was the same editor whose paper had rallied, by means of editorials, against a change at Lawton's old dog pound, where "frightened dogs were pushed into 'squeeze chutes' on their way to less-than-humane deaths, where rats were as large as small cats, and animals were left on weekends in a tin-roofed, completely unventilated building where temperatures soared to over 120 degrees."

I also pointed out that it was obvious that Ralston was lacking in information and knowledge of the seriousness of pet overpopulation and its impact on a community.

I noted that when philosophies do change, or humane advocates propose sensible steps to end the annual national slaughter of our pets, we must battle through ignorance, politics, greed, and private interests, and be labeled, at best, radical or over-reactionary, and, at worst, crazy.

I ended my piece by attempting to convince Mr. Ralston to join forces with us. "Come on, Mr. Ralston. Let's join forces to eliminate the appalling annual slaughter of pets in Lawton and stop the 'pet brouhaha' at city hall once and for all."

Soon thereafter, a no-chain law was passed in Lawton by a majority of members of the City Council. It remains in effect today, however, I can't be certain whether or not it is strongly enforced. It has, however, been replicated by communities throughout the nation.

I WOULD BE remiss not to credit the aforementioned Jeff Wilkinson for his insight into the need for, and value of, no chain laws.

I first became acquainted with Wilkinson, by phone, although I never met him in person. A few years earlier, he had set into place an ordinance banning chaining in Maumelle, and we patterned our ordinance here in Lawton after the one in Maumelle.

Wilkinson was special—one of a small, rare group of animal control officers who was ahead of his time. He told me he didn't believe in eight-to-five animal control and he gives the illusion that he is out twenty-four hours a day. He said if police call at ten o'clock, he goes and gets the animal. "If I'm trapping wild cats, I work until two in the morning. We diligently work on trapping wild cats here," he told me. That is a rarity in most municipal animal control facilities where citizens are left to do that job, as is the case here in Lawton. Jeff Wilkinson was actually concerned about the animals in his care. He knew about pet overpopulation firsthand, and he supported and obtained breeding laws. He epitomized what the field of animal control should really represent—but rarely does.

I spoke to Officer Wilkinson on several occasions back then, and I still have a copy of his poem entitled "Maddie." He called it: "A poem of love from a real life event."

I am not a qualified critic, and I can't comment on Wilkinson's talent as a poet. I can only empathize with the pain he must have been feeling as he penned the following words:

She's a pretty little cat I love,
Her eyes are blue as the sky above. Her fur is soft as a cotton ball,
And white as the winter's snow.

She likes to play with lots of string, And also with her bell that rings.
I pet her and speak softly to her, For in my arms, I hold her.

A friend I have shortly come to meet, She's starting to fall asleep.
A tear I shed for I hate
That from this sleep she shall not awake.

For the fatal dose of drug I gave,
She will never see the break of another day.
A burden, unwanted, and discarded by others, But, loved by me, unlike the others.

Rest in peace, my friend Maddie, For you go unto a better place.
It's sad that you must leave this earth, But never again do I want you to hurt.

This is why I must do what I have done, To protect you for eternity.
Oh, God, how I hate what I must do,
For the mistakes of others, I must undo.

What can we say, as a civilized society, about the pain in the heart of a young, caring animal control officer who just ended the life of a cat called Maddie?

What can we say about the heart of anyone who could allow a dog to die at the end of a metal chain, or a council representative—one of them a veterinarian—who would vote against outlawing that practice?

CHAPTER 37

"There ain't no answer. There ain't gonna be any answer. There never has been an answer. There's your answer." — Gertrude Stein

TWO STEPS FORWARD and one step back. It's not the waltz or the Texas two-step. It's the dance we dance in the ever-frustrating world of animal welfare.

Barely do animal protectionists have time to revel in the success of a newly-enacted law to protect animals only to learn, a few months later, that the pet breeding industry has hired lawyers to challenge the law, and the judge in the case is asking the government's attorney what evidence demonstrates the seriousness of the problem.

What evidence? What evidence demonstrates the seriousness of the problem?

The government's attorney, most likely, knows little or nothing about the problem of pet overpopulation in America. The chance is remote that he has ever, in his life, been in an Oklahoma puppy mill, or any other of the hundreds of breeding shops of horror that blemish the landscape in the remote boondocks of rural America. He has probably never experienced the sight of a rusty metal barrel filled with the bodies of once-healthy dogs and cats who died for a sin no greater than being born. Has he ever even visited a tax-supported animal shelter?

U. S. District Judge Christopher Cooper questioned Justice Department attorney Timothy Johnson about complaints: "What in the record supports the proportionality of the response?" The government's attorney was not up to the question. He concedes to the judge that he doesn't have specific complaints.

The breeders' attorney downplayed the complaint issue saying there had only been a "handful."

Michael Doyle, a writer for the McClatchy Washington Bureau, reported on October 9, 2014, that the Department of Agriculture's licensing and inspection standards imposed in 2013, billed as a crackdown on Internet puppy mills, are being challenged by both dog and cat breeder organizations.

"Chihuahua breeders are snapping at new federal rules that regulate Internet pet dealers. And they're part of a larger pack," Doyle wrote.

This law was like music to the ears of those of us who know, beyond a shadow of a doubt, that puppies and kittens sold on the Internet are, in too many cases, bred in filthy, inhumane surroundings; and contribute overwhelmingly to the overpopulation problem.

An attorney for the breeders, Philip Herbert Hecht, said the Internet rules are "unjustified regulatory overreach . . . a blunderbuss to kill a fly." In all probability, Mr. Hecht also knows nothing of the havoc wreaked by pet breeders who pump out their wares, in massive litters, without conscience nor moral capacity with regard to the negative impact of their actions on animals, and humans, and taxpayers—on all of society.

This law regulating Internet puppy sales is one of the greatest Federal laws to protect animals in recent years. Selling tens of thousands of puppies and kittens on the Internet does not equate to selling gadgets and trinkets on Ebay or Amazon—no matter what pet breeders proclaim to the judge. Puppies and kittens are live, sentient beings who should not be considered commodities.

The bottom line for the pet breeders is just that: The bottom line.

According to Doyle's article, the Obama administration defended the rules as appropriate, and well within the Agriculture Department's authority, and the Humane Society of the United States has gotten involved in support of the new law, declaring that vulnerable animals "will finally get the protection they deserve."

But not if the pet breeding industry has its way. And not if the USDA, and other agencies hold true to their tradition of not aggressively enforcing the laws.

AT ABOUT THE same time the Internet law was being opposed by the pet breeding industry in court, a new dance begins. A call comes from Rose Wilson, Supervisor of Lawton Animal Welfare, with whom we still had a working relationship at that time, who is sharing information that Fort Sill, the military base right under our noses—the one whose name our city council voted to become a part of the name of our city—Lawton-Fort Sill—was adopting out animals in their veterinary and stray facility to the general public, without adhering to either local or state laws regarding neutering and spaying. A phone call confirms they were indeed releasing animals without neutering and spaying because, in the words of an employee there, it makes "adoptions cheaper."

We had worked hard in support of a mandatory neuter/spay law in Lawton that was passed unanimously by council members in 2007. We had served on the Oklahoma Legislative Committee in 1986 to help pass the Dog and

Cat Sterilization Act that requires all adopted pets be neutered or spayed in communities with populations over 10,000 in Oklahoma.

The military base was not only ignoring the laws, but competing with humane groups by adopting animals cheaper to the general public because they were not required to comply with the law.

We start to make phone calls. Finally, someone from the Pentagon in Washington, D.C. calls and tells me he will check on all this, and get back to us in a couple of days. Six weeks later, we've heard nothing. We call council members who don't like it either, but, of course, can't be negatively vocal about anything concerning Fort Sill. So it's going to be up to us to write the letters, to make the calls, to create controversy; to make ourselves unpopular–even reviled; because sometimes it seems we are the only ones paying attention to these things.

Many of the surrounding no-kill rescue and adoption groups are generally unhappy as it is with a recently passed Oklahoma House Bill 1359, the Commercial Pet Breeders and Animal Shelter Licensing Act, which helps regulate shelters, or those who house 10 or more homeless dogs and/or cats to ensure they are cared for properly.

The groups see the bill as an annoyance that interferes with their daily adoption routines. It is overseen by the Oklahoma Department of Agriculture, and requires pet breeders and rescue organizations to be licensed and inspected in efforts to reduce the number of cruelty charges—among breeders and rescue organizations.

Because we house a few homeless dogs and cats, we signed up the Animal Birth Control Clinic, even though, as a veterinary clinic, we were exempt from the law. We wanted to show support.

After we mailed our application and our check for $200.00, we were inspected by a USDA veterinarian/inspector and received our license. It was license number 0001. We obviously were the first in the state to get a license.

House Bill 1359 takes baby steps in the long walk to the finish line of pet overpopulation in Oklahoma, as does the Federal Internet law; but every little bit helps. Too many of the no-kill groups, however, can't be bothered to embrace measures to eliminate pet overpopulation—at its core.

God knows everyone is busy. Adoptions are a critical part of the multi-faceted approach to solutions. But while we are busy rescuing and fostering and neutering and spaying and vaccinating and adopting, breeders and irresponsible pet owners continue to grind out litter after litter from tired old dogs and cats—in a nation almost completely unfettered with pet breeding restrictions, without which the killing will never end and the vicious cycle will continue to repeat itself.

In 1992, we had a licensing law that was an early version of today's mandatory spay/neuter laws. It was a miracle, a real coup, at that point in history, that such a small city had such an aggressive law—one of the few of its kind in the nation. But it was never once enforced, due to politics, and an animal welfare supervisor who didn't fight to enforce it. Non-enforcement of good laws is a big part of the massive pet overpopulation problem.

That neuter/spay law in our city, the Bat Permit, that passed in 2007 by a unanimous vote of city council? No sooner was the law placed into the city code, when it was threatened by a newly- elected council member who thought the law was too "radical" because his friend paid a hefty fine for allowing his unneutered pit bull to run at large; and another council member's friend from a nearby rural town had been caught selling puppies in Lawton without a permit and were challenging the law. So there we were-back at city hall, on two separate occasions, fighting for the law all over again. We persevered and the law is intact even though it was tweaked to render it less effective.

It's been that way from the beginning. Whether it's the ongoing effort to reduce the killing of dogs and cats through massive neuter/spay efforts; or the heartfelt desire for a humanely-operated city animal shelter; or laws to regulate pet breeding and protect animals; or begging authorities for prosecution of obvious cruelty cases—all become battles in which we dance the dance. Two steps forward and one step back. Sometimes the dance is reversed. One step forward and two steps back.

We, at least, want to believe that humane societies and others who care about animals are in our corner—if they are not openly fighting the battle with us, they are silently supporting us.

Then someone tells us to go online and read the Declaration of the No Kill Movement in the United States—those people who believe that adoptions, and adoptions only, will somehow win the war on the mass killing of millions of dogs and cats. And, as we read the Declaration, we gasp in disbelief that not only does this movement call for the repeal of some sound animal control laws, their Declaration doesn't even mention the words neuter or spay. Then our angst mode rises to just below the explosion level as we discover that people in that movement are telling the world online there is no pet overpopulation problem in America. That it is all just a myth! On what planet are these people living? We already knew that the ASPCA never mentions neuter/spay in their TV ads and is against mandatory neuter/spay laws.

Then, momentarily, we allow ourselves to think that maybe this is all there is. Maybe this is all there's ever going to be. Adopt. Abandon. Rescue. Foster. Repeat. Or the other scenario: Adopt. Abandon. Euthanize. Repeat.

And those of us dancing the dance, feeling hopeless and defeated, wring our hands in despair and cry to the Heavens: "There ain't no answer. There ain't gonna be any answer. There never has been an answer.

Ultimately, a calm ensues. And the dance continues.

THE CHIHUAHUA BREEDERS who are "snapping" at the new federal rules that regulate Internet pet dealers, would never admit they are part of the larger problem of animal suffering and death.

Neither would Martha Stewart. I caught the world-famous domestic diva on a late night talk show where the subject was—before I switched the channel—her male Chow Chow dog Genghis Khan II. Ms. Stewart, looking perky for her age, was all smiles. She joyfully shared with the show's host, Seth Meyers, the news that her dog was waiting for a female dog in Pennsylvania to come into "you know what," as she described it; and they were going to make puppies.

The idea of driving a dog across several states to have sex with another dog for the purpose of bringing more dogs into an already dog-crowded world was repulsive to me. I try to visualize it—two dog owners discussing their dogs having sex. How does that work? Do they watch the process? All I can think about is that these humans are pimps. They are actually pimping their dogs.

The very next evening, Tia Torres of the reality show *Pit Bulls and Parolees* was a guest on *The Daily Show* with comedian Jon Stewart, who, obviously, is a pit bull advocate. I have watched the *Pit Bulls and Parolees* show maybe a half dozen times, and am impressed with what they do. Torres doesn't just talk the talk. She walks the walk. She doesn't just go to animal shelters and pick up her pit bulls. She rescues pitiful dogs from dangerous situations; and, from what can be determined from the television show, she thoroughly screens potential adopters. I was, however, discouraged to hear they are now caring for more than 400 homeless pit bull dogs.

Contrast the difference. Martha Stewart on the *Seth Meyers Show* beaming about breeding her Chow Chow; and within twenty-four hours, Tia Torres is on *The Daily Show* discussing the hardships of her life rescuing and caring for 400 abandoned dogs—that should never have been born.

What's wrong with this picture?

ALTA, UTAH, HAS the answer; and I'm not so sure they even know the question. The Town of Alta may have, unwittingly, stumbled onto the answer to pet overpopulation problems in the rest of the country.

The tiny ski resort town, nestled in the Wasatch National Forest on the outskirts of Salt Lake City, is a protected watershed area that supplies drinking water to Salt Lake Valley. It has a colorful history, including mining, and boasts home to the second chairlift in United States history.

According to the town's website, because dog waste contains bacteria and parasites that can make drinking water unsafe, the Town of Alta has a licensing process that permits a very limited number of dogs within the town limits. The licensees must comply with other pet restrictions and requirements. Owners of property in Alta have first rights to licenses.

My plastic tubs contained a 2006 Associated Press article about dog licensing in Alta. "Every January when dog licenses come up for renewal in this ski town, dog lovers go wild with anticipation," the article stated. "They start counting the dogs that have died or moved away with their owners, hoping a few licenses will be available."

At the time the article was written, the town limited the number of dogs to 12 percent of the human population, which in Alta at that time was 370. That figure allowed only 42 dog licenses to be issued. Today, 15 percent of the 383 full-time residents are allowed licenses to own dogs.

Alta mayors admit it's the worst issue they have to deal with. Residents are obviously scrambling to latch onto a more-valuable-than-gold dog license.

One is required to purchase a temporary license even on a visit to Alta, Utah, with a dog. Temporary licenses are $75 for a stay of less than two weeks; and, for more than two weeks, the fee is $125 for a neutered dog and $150 for an unsterilized dog. This doesn't always set well with visitors. Fees are also hefty for the dogs of permanent residents.

I spoke to Kate Black, city recorder for the Town of Alta, who has been at her job for over 40 years. She admitted their dog ordinances are more comprehensive than perhaps any in the country. "We have strict animal ordinances, including leash laws and fecal matter waste laws."

I quizzed her about whether they have an animal control department, or even an animal shelter.

Nope. No need for an animal shelter or animal control in Alta, Utah. "Police enforce the animal ordinances," she told me. "Ninety eight percent of the residents play by the rules. We have very few issues at all."

Wow! Almost no animal issues at all! I think I want to move there. A community with no strays! No cruelties! A place where there is no need for week-end adopt-a-thons; a place where people line up and wait to be able to own a dog, instead of dogs being lined up in euthanasia rooms waiting to be killed!

Black admitted they have been called every name in the book for their strict animal ordinances.

"Totally ridiculous." That's what Maureen Hill-Hauch, executive director of the American Dog Owners Association, said of the law in the 2006 Associated Press article.

"No other town limits dogs. How can people live without dogs?" she said. "It sounds like a total and complete violation of a person's civil rights. How dare they?"

Yeah, Maureen. How dare they? How dare there be any community in this country where a citizen can go to bed on a cold night without having to think about the dogs and cats who are outside in a blizzard starving to death. And they are out there! Trust me. They are out there! And just who does Alta, Utah, think they are, anyway, to totally have no use for an animal shelter where normal activities include killing healthy dogs and cats at a cost of hundreds of thousands of dollars to local taxpayers. Yes, Maureen. How dare they?

It goes without saying there are no pet breeders in this tiny pristine community, that is reportedly going green. I didn't ask Kate Black if there was a requirement that all dogs be neutered or spayed. That goes without saying, too. Do you think you would be able to retain your coveted dog license if you showed up at city hall requesting eight more licenses for a litter of puppies?

I don't think so!

Alta, Utah, could be a model for the rest of the nation if we want to end pet overpopulation, and the animal suffering and killing that goes along with it.

Regulate, restrict and tax pet breeding! And strictly enforce those laws!

There's your answer!

CHAPTER 38

"Usually, stories on the subject of animal abandonment show a cute little cocker, panting lovingly into the camera, begging for adoption. What is left unsaid is the consequence of public indifference to the problem: a grim scenario of death and incineration, a scenario that is virtually never discussed, never written about, never photographed."
— John Dorschner, *The Miami Herald*, from See Spot Die

"LINDA," I SAID, "This is what people want to hear. Seriously. Who would not love to read this?"

Linda and I were driving home from taking care of some business at the Animal Birth Control Clinic, where I had picked up a copy of the Pet Gazette, the publication of the local current humane society. I was reading to Linda as she was driving.

That day had been a particularly busy one. Linda and I had interviewed a potential new veterinarian interested in performing an additional day of neuters and spays at the clinic. The clinic also had been slammed that day with an overabundance of large and/or pregnant female dogs. Linda instructs our employees to overbook to counter inevitable and historical no-shows, some of which have been booked for free surgery. On this particular surgery day, however, everyone and his dog—and cat—had shown up.

The twelve-page humane society newsletter was well designed, in full color, on heavy stock paper with a considerable number of business card advertisements, an indication of support from the community. Stories of animals adopted, and those waiting for adoption, were written with flair, the work of an obviously talented writer. This was the humane society that we had formed back in 1986 for the purpose of contracting with the city to operate the animal shelter. During my exile to the Sonoran Desert (discussed in a later chapter) Linda had turned that organization and the IRS 501(c)3 non-profit status to a new group of people, along with our funny-looking doggie fund-raising banks.

I found myself intrigued with each animal's biography in the Pet Gazette. Ziggarilli's story was featured on the cover with colorful pictures of what appeared to be a small Yorkie or Llaso Apso playing in a patch of green English Ivy.

"My name is Ziggarilli," the article began. "My friends call me Ziggi. Earlier in my life, I wanted to join the Air Force and soar through the air. I just love their uniforms and the ladies just love guys in uniform. I would be a commander of course. I like being in charge. I could hear myself saying, 'Commander Ziggi to Base; come in please. I am at Zero 695 altitude with 20% visibility; request landing instructions.' 'Roger!' Coming in from the west low and slow . . . over and out." Sigh . . . that would be so exciting.

"Then on the other hand, I would really like being on the stage singing and dancing. I would be stunning in a gold lame suit with a diamond studded scarf. I would not sing any songs that were in bad taste . . . such as 'Hound Dog,' 'How Much is that Doggie in the Window?' or 'Who Let the Dogs out?' How crude! My style would be much more sophisticated. I was talking to a squirrel that lives next door about my totally exciting plans; he told me I should chill out and relax. Relax!? He doesn't know the meaning of the word. He is always rushing around frantically looking for his nuts or hiding his nuts, burying his nuts or digging up his nuts. I don't get it. I am just happy hanging out with my human dreaming of all the things that are possible."

I surprised myself that I was able to make it through the lengthy fluff piece. I think it was a welcome distraction from the bad news of the day, i.e. learning about the military's bad adoption policies, and the news that pet breeders were challenging the Agriculture Department's Internet law.

On the next page, I saw Jo Jo and Lillie pictured in a pile of laundry, attesting to their love of nesting in clean clothes. On the same page, was George, the human Gentle Giant, who, the article said, "has cared for more cats than most of us see in a lifetime." George is a neuter/spay advocate and a friend and client of the Animal Birth Control Clinic, as are all the humane society members.

I flipped on over to page four to read of the astonishing case of Scooter, one of a litter of eight kittens. Scooter was born with a condition called "Manx Syndrome." In utero, his spinal column didn't fully develop, and his back legs were badly mangled. A veterinarian had removed the poor kitten's back legs, and, according to this amazing story, he does great on those front legs, and it didn't take Scooter long to develop fans on the Internet from all over the world.

"A year later, he's a fully grown cat now who has still not learned to like that diaper!" the story revealed.

All twelve pages of this humane society publication were filled with wonderful, heart-warming stories about animals finding homes—or at least a foster home.

Telly was a two-time (so far) loser, who was left outside by his owners with very little food or water. Lonely and hungry, he made his way out of the back yard and ran away. He was picked up by a stranger and taken to an animal shelter where he was once again adopted. Telly's luck, however, was no better this time around. Once again Telly was left alone without food or water or that longed-for gentle hugging and petting. He wandered the streets again. He then went into foster care yet again.

I had a thing about Telly. His story bothered me—a lot. I can't say why. For some reason, I was having flashbacks of the old, white Poodle, sitting terrified in that horrible city animal shelter twenty-eight years ago. Did I have room for one more dog in my home? There are seven now. Am I becoming a collector?

I needed to avoid another layer of emotional baggage, so I made a call to Donna, an active member of the humane society. Donna is the Cat Lady Supreme with the organization. She is in our clinic, or some other veterinary clinic, with cats galore almost every day.

I asked Donna about Telly. I learned he is a purebred Chihuahua; that he had been adopted from the nearby Stephens County Humane Society (was this a screened adoption?); that he was super thin and often kept on a chain outside, even though that is illegal in Lawton, but animal control was never able to catch the owners in the act. I learned that a concerned neighbor was able to get possession of the little Chihuahua by offering his owners forty dollars; and that he then was placed in a Lawton Humane Society foster home. Donna told me Telly had since been adopted by someone in Fletcher, Oklahoma, about twenty-five minutes from Lawton.

I begged Donna to call and check on Telly. I had become obsessed with Telly's plight. She reported back to me that she was certain Telly—who now has a new name—has a wonderful home with people who love him dearly. It's about time. The helpless little dog has been shuffled from foster home to semi-permanent home to animal shelter—and back again. I pray to God it's permanent this time.

Finding homes for dogs and cats is the number one priority with humane societies and rescue groups here in Lawton and across America. Some of their active, well-meaning, overworked, members will not abort a pregnant dog or cat—as a side effect of a spay.

As for me, I have been programmed to be distrustful of humans when it comes to adopting animals. It is only common sense to believe that a large percentage of the animals who end up in animal shelters are the same ones who were adopted on a whim at a local adoption event.

In the words of Meryl Streep at the end of the movie *Doubt*: "I have doubts. I have such doubts."

MY CRITICISM OF the no-kill movement should not—by any stretch of the imagination—be interpreted as approval, or acceptance, of killing as a means of dealing with an overabundance of unwanted pets. I have railed against the senselessness of that practice by whatever means has been available to me since I first learned there are more dogs and cats in America than there are people to care for them. I will take to my grave the emotional scars I carry from witnessing too many cruelties, too much suffering, and too many euthanasias—all of which are the result of pet breeding.

My viewpoint, and my approach, has been that to end the killing, we must turn off the faucet.

My complaint with the no-kill movement is that the faucet is still running; and handing out buckets of water does not diminish the flood. In PETA's words, the kittens are still floating down the river.

I agree completely that we must promote adoptions—placing a stigma on buying pets from breeders and pet shops. We have promoted shelter adoptions since day one.

Shelter workers also need to step up to the plate and shoulder some of the responsibility. I believe when you get caught up in the euthanasia trap, one of two things happens: You either accept it as the manner in which we handle uncontrolled and unrestricted pet breeding in our society; or you clench your fists and vow to change it. Shelter workers need to clench their fists—along with the rest of us.

What would happen if the millions of no-kill advocates across the nation would spend just half the time—just half—they spend at PetSmart, and other adoption sites, or driving pets to homes across the country, demanding local, state, and federal government agencies enact strict breeding laws—with no loopholes whatsoever—all across America?

What if all of us, across this nation, who are dedicated to this cause—this mind-boggling, time-consuming, energy-draining, gut-wrenching cause—simply announced that we will no longer do it! No longer will we quietly clean house for the breeders and irresponsible pet owners in this country.

No longer will we kill the victims and then sweep the dirty little killing secrets under the rug. No longer will we provide foster homes, or humane society shelters, or tax-supported shelters. How much longer are we willing to tolerate trailer loads of corpses headed to a county landfill or fiery incinerators burning the beautiful bodies of innocent dogs and cats?

What if we refuse to continue to hold garage and bake sales, and plead for grants and donations; and do such weird things as try to operate a bingo hall? Why should we use our own money to provide for the needs of animals we did not bring into this world?

How much longer should we be willing to chase the strays; trap and neuter; neuter and spay; cry; sometimes see our relationships, our marriages, our bank accounts, and even our health ruined—as well as our reputations?

What if we demand laws to control pet breeding to the extent that supply equals demand—where no dog or cat is homeless, or neglected, or killed, simply because we have tip-toed around the pet breeding industry for decades?

When do we say enough is enough?

What if we simply told our local, state and federal governments: We want our lives back!

If we are to be the humane nation we've convinced ourselves we are, then we're going to have to run upstream to see, as PETA has suggested, who's throwing kittens in the water—and finally stop them!

CHAPTER 39

"It is a greater sin to be cruel to the dumb creation, almost, than it is to be unkind to human beings, as the latter can complain, and have laws to protect them, but the former often have no redress." — T. Augustus Forbes

"DEAR MR. PRESIDENT," the letter began. "I am writing to you because I need help. I've tried everything I know of, maybe you can help me."

The letter was dated February 20, 1989. The president was George H. W. Bush.

"Please find enclosed with this letter a copy of my story and pictures that I sent to all the public officials, congressmen, senators, and agencies. They all seemed like they wanted to help, but the laws tied their hands, and misjustice, (sic) I feel has been done.

"Mr. Spann was arrested on January 17, 1989, on 4 felony counts of pet cruelty; but then a few days later the charges were dropped because the pet cruelty laws were written in the 1800's in Oklahoma, and don't help animals much if any.

"Now Mr. Spann is trying to get his dogs back. You see an animal lover— Dolores (sic) Delluomo and some others went to Spann's "dog farm" and took 28 of the sickest, weakest dogs and gave them shelter, food, and vet care. One died—it couldn't be saved. Now the remaining 27 dogs are healthy and Mr. Spann wants them back. I'm so afraid of what will happen to them if he does.

"We must change these laws so that legal officials can do their jobs and stop this from happening anymore. Animals give so much to us humans, can't we at least give them enough protection to be treated right?

"I thank you for taking time to read this Mr. President. My local TV station is going to air this story soon. You two are my last hopes—but I won't give up. I just can't in my heart."

The letter was signed: "Respectfully yours, Daniel S. Kingston, Sr."

I never met Daniel S. Kingston of Dingman's Ferry, Pennsylvania, nor do I recall ever even speaking to him on the phone.

I do, however, have a file folder full of correspondence between Mr. Kingston and an astonishing number of government agencies, politicians, media, and humane organizations from whom he had sought help.

I learned of Kingston's dilemma when Holly Hazard of the Doris Day Animal League contacted me, as president of the humane society. Kingston appealed to the Doris Day Animal League on December 5, 1988.

"This is a letter of concern, statement and fact about a hunting dog I purchased from a man through the mail, recently," the letter began.

"I first called Al Spann on Tuesday night, November 8th after seeing his ad for hunting dogs for sale in the October issue of *Sports Afield Magazine*. I told him I was looking for a bird dog, somewhat trained already and he said he had an 18-month-old Brittany-English Setter mix who had a great nose and pointed birds well. I asked him if the dog was in good shape - he said yes. I asked him what kind of guarantee he gave and he said the dog was everything he said it was. The dog's name was Bullet.

"I sent him a money order for $550—the next morning—Wednesday, November 9th for the dog.

"Five hundred dollars for Bullet, $50.00 for the shipping crate," Kingston wrote. "He sent the dog out from Oklahoma on Wednesday morning, November 16th and I picked up the dog with a friend Frank Gallo, whose address and phone I will leave at the end also, for he will testify what he saw also at Newark airport, Newark, N.J. on that same night.

"I couldn't believe what I saw come out of that shipping crate. It was a dog much older than 18 months, with its bones sticking out all over, thick mucus coming from its nose and mouth, a puffy face, and diarrhea. I was sick and very disturbed that someone could treat an animal like this, much less sell one. I couldn't refuse the animal for return shipping for I felt it would die in flight.

"I thought if I fed the dog well and kept him warm he might get better, but he got worse and I got scared and took him to the vet on November 21st. The vet's report is enclosed. I called Al Spann and said what kind of dog did you send me? He said I've got 50 dogs and I can't afford to feed them protein food; but this dog was treated, neglected, much more than that, I could see and so did the vet.

"With all we could do, the dog, my dog, died on Thanksgiving day - eight days after I received him. I buried him in a sunny spot behind my house, tears in my eyes. I called Al Span again and asked him what he wanted to do about it. He said the best he could do was to sell me another one half price. Can you believe it?? What gaul! (Sic.)

"I feel I can't let this man keep treating his animals like this, and ripping people off either for I feel this is mail fraud. I am going to do everything I legally can to stop him. It just isn't right.

"I would like some response, personal response from this letter. I want this guy's dogs checked out, and taken away if need be, and last of all and least of all I'd like my reimbursement for the dog and my other bills associated with this case. Thank you."

Kingston signed the letter "Very concerned and upset. Sincerely, Daniel S. Kingston. His bill for the dog, the crate, shipping and vet came to $858.68.

THE OFFICE OF the Regional Chief Inspector of the U. S. Postal Service called it a private civil matter "since there is insufficient basis to begin a mail fraud investigation."

The Office of the Attorney General of Pennsylvania, to whom Kingston appealed, suggested he accept Spann's settlement offer of a new dog for half price.

The Federal Trade Commission told him his complaint was being added to their computerized reporting system; and that it is important for them to know of problems consumers are experiencing.

Kingston reported his story to Senators Charles Lemmond and Jeannette Reibman of Pennsylvania; Rep. Dave McCurdy, Senator Don Nickels, Governor Henry Bellmon and the attorney general of Oklahoma. He contacted the Humane Society of the United States; WNEP TV Channel 16 Action News; ASPCA; the Doris Day Animal League; *Sports Afield Magazine*; as well as other hunting and dog magazines; Action line in New York, New York News; and the Oklahoma veterinarian who provided the health certificate with the dog. Of all those contacted, he received no real help from anyone other than the Doris Day Animal League.

The Volunteers for Animal Welfare of Oklahoma City had received complaints about the dogs at Spann's facility. Lynda Powell, president of the group, said they went to the site and found one of the "worst things I have seen in some ten years since I began working with our organization."

Powell's group took four of the worst dogs immediately to a veterinarian with permission of the local sheriff.

In an article written by Bryan Martin of the Daily Oklahoman, Powell was quoted as saying, "We saw about twenty dogs four of which were terribly emaciated. Others were thin. Buckets of water were frozen and black and obviously contaminated. Some food scattered around the pens was covered with feces." Spann was arraigned, the article said, but released from jail on a personal recognizance bond. "An investigation was launched after two animal groups received complaints from people who had arranged to buy bird dogs. The complaints surfaced through the Volunteers for Animal Welfare of Oklahoma City and the Lawton Humane Society."

Holly Hazard, Executive Director of the Doris Day Animal League in Washington, D. C. responded to Kingston's desperate appeal for help. She then contacted us.

"DO YOU HAVE puppies for sale," Linda asked the bird dog farmer. "I'd like to see your puppies." After being contacted by Hazard, Linda and Dayman, and Dan and I had driven the seventy-five miles to Norman to assess the situation.

It took us what seemed like forever to find the place. It was typical of an Oklahoma puppy mill—a nasty place, hidden from the world, in the middle of nowhere.

On pulling up to the facility, we could see dogs in individual pens with little or no real shelter. The dog breeder met Linda and Dayman down by the entry to the property. We decided Linda would pose as a buyer. The man, who we later learned was Spann, was vague about whether or not he even had any puppies. He was adamant about selling one of the older dogs instead.

"No," Linda insisted. "My husband likes to train his own dogs so I need a puppy. He has a birthday soon and I want to get him a puppy."

Reluctantly, Spann pointed to a hillside behind the dog pens. As Linda and Dayman were in pursuit of their bird dog puppy, Dan and I were nosing around the property. The stench was horrendous and the dogs were in pitiful condition. Linda was not allowed to see the puppies on that occasion.

We returned to Lawton, and after numerous phone calls to the sheriff in that county, we received a call that there was a warrant for Spann's arrest, and as soon as he was in custody, we could seize the dogs.

The task that lay ahead of us was immense. Our facility was in no way large enough to house that many dogs; but we had to get them out of the horrific conditions under which they were living.

We panicked. But we had faced the impossible before, and usually beat the odds. We gathered up as many people and as many vehicles as possible. My oldest son, Monty, who lives in Oklahoma City, met us there to help. It was imperative we get there to get the dogs before Spann was released from jail.

It was the middle of the winter, and by the time we arrived in Norman, it was dark. Here we were on this strange property, grabbing up dogs as fast as possible, not knowing if we were going to be bitten—or shot. I do remember Linda was "packing heat" as she always did on these occasions.

Luckily, we encountered no opposition to taking the dogs. The place seemed deserted. Thank God no one had to "say hello" to Linda's little friend. I'm not sure I would have trusted her aim.

Linda finally found the puppies. They were sick and thin, and the same was true of the mother dogs. They were in metal barrels cut in half and lined with hay, but had no shelter from the elements.

We loaded dogs into stock trailers and automobiles. Linda was with me in my station wagon sitting in the back compartment holding one of the larger bird dogs. Some of these dogs, who had had very little, or no, socialization, appeared to have psychological problems. The one particular dog Linda was holding would constantly lunge, trying to get away. Another person, sitting next to Linda, was holding a dog with the same problem; and keeping them separated was a challenge.

A litter of puppies in the front seat of the vehicle kept falling off between the seat and the car door. I was driving, but I kept trying to pull them back up onto the seat.

If the situation hadn't been so tragic, it could have been a comedy skit from an episode of Saturday Night Live.

We literally have physical scars from these types of episodes, as well as emotional ones. Sitting on the hard floor in the back of the station wagon did a number on Linda's back. And if that didn't do her in, then she almost finished destroying her back when we arrived at the clinic. As she and I lifted a large stainless steel kennel, in which we had transported a large male pointer, out of the vehicle in which it had been transported, her back went completely out that time.

To this day, she still has back problems from this rescue, but, she says, "it was well worth the effort—and pain—to see those dogs out of that horrible place." That was not the first—nor would it be the last— heavy dog kennel, or trap, we would lift over the years, bad backs or not.

The next night, a young woman, who was a humane society volunteer, and I drove back to the dog farm, rushed onto the property, and hastily gathered up the last three or four of the dogs for which we had not had room the previous evening. As I look back, I have to wonder if we were in our right minds. I don't know if I'd have the guts to do that today.

We had made arrangements with a kennel that was on the outskirts of Lawton to house the dogs until we could figure out something. My youngest son, Paul, had a small construction company at the time, and he built a building with runs, on the land right beside the Animal Birth Control Clinic.

IN THE MEANTIME, Holly Hazard was making the case to the USDA that Spann's dogs fell under the protection of the Animal Welfare Act, pressuring the government to act in this case. The USDA was, however, anything but helpful—which came as no surprise.

On March 1, 1989, Hazard, an attorney, wrote a response to a letter from USDA agent Pat Allen. "My interpretation of the law as it relates to this case is different from that of the Department as written in your letter."

Dr. Allen, a veterinarian, was claiming there was a question as to whether or not the Spann dogs come under the "retail" exemption for dog dealers.

"In your letter, you state that it has been Department policy not to regulate persons selling dogs and cats on a retail basis," wrote Hazard.

"While I understand that the Act does not include retail stores . . . I don't believe that it is a matter of debate that he is not operating a 'retail pet store.'

"It is significant that Chairman Weicker of the Senate Committee that passed the amendments to the bill in 1976 disclosed that his reasons for initiating some of the changes in the Act were that he had received a letter from a 'lady in Stanford, Connecticut who had had some German Shepherds shipped to her from the mid-west which dogs arrived dead.' Interestingly, this is essentially the same situation which Mr. Kingston finds himself in, over ten years later. The response of the Department to this is that the dogs in question are not covered under the Animal Welfare Act."

The USDA was also claiming it was questionable as to whether hunting dogs were covered under the law.

"With reference to the question of hunting dogs being covered, I find it astounding that the Department has taken the position that Congress 'gave no clear indication as to their intent in regulating such activities . . .' I draw your attention to the 1976 amendments to the Federal Animal Welfare Act in which the definition of dealer was changed to include specifically 'any person who sells . . . or . . . who delivers for transportation . . . any dog for hunting . . . purposes.' The definition of 'animal' was also changed in 1976 to 'clarify the fact that the term dog means all dogs including those used for hunting . . . purposes.'"

Hazard accused the Department of Agriculture as giving the Animal Welfare Act the lack of priority which has been apparent since its inception. "This disappointment takes a frustrating turn when clear evidence of animal suffering and cruelty are brought to the attention of U.S.D.A. investigators by concerned citizens and still the Department finds excuses not to act."

Most of us in animal welfare—who know and care—have been aware, for years, that the USDA has been a joke when it comes to enforcement of the Animal

Welfare Act. Several years ago, the television show *20/20* did an expose of the USDA's blatant "turning a blind eye" to the cruelties. One USDA veterinarian/investigator was actually operating her own puppy mill at the time.

Hazard wrote a letter addressed to me and the Humane Society of Lawton-Comanche County the same day she wrote to Dr. Allen of the USDA. It included a check for $750.00.

"I hope that this is helpful in providing some assistance in caring for the dogs currently under your care.

"I want you to know how much I appreciate your willingness to become involved in this case. I know that we are all inundated with requests to do just one more thing for the animals. Had you not been able to help in this case, it is extremely unlikely I could have done anything from Washington and the animals that are now out of that situation would still be with Mr. Spann," she wrote.

"I hope that the knowledge of this is as heartening to you as it is to me. I understand that your efforts are far from over. As you know, if there is anything further I can do to help on the Oklahoma front, please let me know. As I get more information from the bureaucrats in Washington I will certainly keep you informed."

We appreciated the letter and the check from Hazard, but it was a drop in the bucket compared to what we had spent to rescue and care for those dogs.

"Your contribution was a lifesaver," I responded to Hazard's letter on April 7th. "The veterinarian bill was in excess of $1,000, and the kennel bill was right around $2,000. We have now moved the dogs (all but three who are still being boarded at the other kennel) over to our facility, which resulted in an additional expenditure of over $5,000 to build a small kennel on our shelter property. As we have room, we move each Spann dog into our facility, as I worry about the security of the new facility.

"Although we hear rumblings of Spann suing for the return of the dogs, nothing has transpired to date. I hope he's faking. At any rate, we are seriously considering starting to neuter and spay the dogs and offering them for adoption, as our kennels are bulging at the seams with dogs. We have about twice as many dogs as we should have and I worry about the welfare of the animals, although we have a very nice facility, and lots of love for each and every one of them."

"I hope you are continuing to pursue the matter with the Department of Agriculture. Frankly, I don't know what those people do!"

INASMUCH AS HAZARD was related to Doris Day and in constant contact with her, I took shameless advantage of the opportunity. I shared with her my delusions of grandeur; my visions of awakening an uninformed America to the disgrace of pet overpopulation; and the suffering of animals in breeding facilities such as the Spann operation in Norman, Oklahoma.

"Again, Holly, talk to Ms. Day about the possibility of some sort of national telethon for animal welfare," I wrote. "I know she has the contacts. We will do anything and everything we can on this end, and behind the scenes to make something of that magnitude work. I do believe it is going to take a genuine grass roots movement to truly change this country for our animals. People are just not knowledgeable about the truth."

I shared with her my thoughts about flying to Vegas to talk to Casino owners/ managers to see if there would be any interest in putting together something like an animal welfare telethon on the subject of pet overpopulation and puppy mills like Spann's.

"Interested in accompanying me?" I asked. Bert Parks would be a great MC. I understand Paul McCartney's house is a mess with animals. You know, dog doo on the Persian rugs. Surely, the many stars that love animals would get involved. Isn't it time?"

I included a postscript and copy of a letter to the Prudential Insurance Company we had written in an attempt to convince them to select Linda in a competition to recognize employees who perform outstanding volunteer service in their communities.

"Linda certainly fills the bill," I wrote. "We desperately need the money involved in the award." We asked Hazard to put in a good word for us if she was contacted by Prudential.

Unfortunately, Linda did not win the award. My guess would be it went to someone who was involved with human social causes. Some have the wrong impression of those of us in animal welfare. They see us helping animals to the exclusion of human beings.

One thing, however, is certain. When our phone rings—and it has rang non-stop over the years—it is never a dog or a cat, or any other animal, on the other end of the line.

It is always a human being who is asking for our help!

WE HAD THE Spann dogs for months. They ate all they wanted of good quality food; had warm beds on which to rest their tired bodies; were cool in the summer and warm in the winter; had room to run; and they were loved by all of us.

Eventually, we were able to adopt several of them to people with whom we felt comfortable enough to do so.

I know we were unable to adopt them all.

I relate this twenty-seven-year-old story to illustrate how government has done so little over the years to protect animals in spite of laws put into place for that purpose. Kingston was told there was nothing that could be done against Spann for mistreatment of his dogs because the animal cruelty laws in Oklahoma were inadequate. That is not true. Oklahoma has good anti-cruelty laws and they were in place in 1988. Getting those laws enforced has been the problem. Many in law enforcement don't even realize the laws are on the books; while others just don't give a damn!

Bird dogs are some of the most loving dogs—and make some of the best pets—on earth.

Because they are considered working dogs, they generally get a really bad rap. To think they would be exempt from any laws that protect animals is unconscionable.

The stories of the abused and neglected bird dogs took their places in my plastic tub of memories, along with the greyhounds, and hundreds of others, for which I still—to this day—carry an ache in my heart.

Although this is an old story, if anyone, including the no-kill groups who deny the reality of pet overpopulation, believes it is not happening today in puppy mills all over the Midwest, then I have a bridge in London—or Lake Havasu City, Arizona, or wherever the hell that bridge is now—I'd like to sell them.

CHAPTER 40

"I don't know how to save the world. I don't have the answers or The Answer. I hold no secret knowledge as to how to fix the mistakes of generations past and present. I only know that without compassion and respect for all of Earth's inhabitants, none of us will survive—nor will we deserve to." — Leonard Peltier, Imprisoned Native American Activist

IN 1990, AFTER five years of frantically promoting neutering and spaying by every means available, we weren't satisfied with our progress. We had hoped to see a greater reduction in animal euthanasias at the city shelter, which, actually, had been reduced between forty and fifty percent. That still meant, however, that somewhere around 4000 to 4500 animals were still senselessly dying in our city—not to mention the strays in the county where I live.

The fact that we are a transient military community didn't help, although we neuter and spay huge numbers of pets belonging to military families.

By this point, my own passion for the plight of unwanted pets had become almost hopelessly entangled with frustration and pain. Linda and I, our employees, our veterinarians—so many—had toiled "hands-on" for years at great personal expense, and emotional exhaustion, in what was appearing to be an almost hopeless battle against pet overpopulation.

I was, and still am, increasingly angry at irresponsible pet owners who refuse, or are just too lazy and indifferent to have their pets neutered or spayed—even if it is offered to them for free.

I was, and still am, angry at the hobby and back-porch breeders, and puppy millers, who dump on society and leave, in their insatiable quest for profits, a trail of animal suffering and death that is impossible for overworked humanitarians and shelter workers to clean up—not to mention the tremendous burden animal shelters and animal problems place on a community.

Perhaps, most of all, however, I was, and still am, angry at the large—and rich—national organizations who have tiptoed around the pet breeding industry for decades.

How much longer, I was thinking in my despair, can we, as a nation, look into the trusting eyes of innocent pets destined for the euthanasia needle, or less humane deaths, and accept it as the solution for uncontrolled breeding—and still call ourselves humane?

How much longer should we endure the sight of the dead and mangled bodies of this nation's pets along highways, county roads, and city streets?

We had gained control of our deplorable city animal shelter, cleaned it up, helped set good policies in place, and because we realized sheltering and euthanasia were not the answers we were seeking, gave it back. Years later, unfortunately, the battle for a humanely-run animal shelter would have to be fought all over again with an outcome that was stranger than fiction.

At that time, although veterinarians had fought hard against licensing of any kind, we won our battle for general licensing, and a litter permit ordinance, which was not once enforced.

About the time these events were taking place in Lawton, a national Animal Rights Movement was sweeping across the country.

Animal rights activists were dousing fur coats with red paint to simulate blood, in protest of killing animals for fur. Consumers were being asked to boycott tuna because fishermen were catching dolphins in their nets. Ivory was not to be purchased due to poaching of elephants, and whaling and the killing of seals and sea lions were also big issues.

These were all good causes. But what about the killing of millions of excess, unwanted pets, and the fact that there were no restrictions on pet breeding?

We began to ask ourselves hard questions.

Why, we were asking, wasn't the shelter establishment taking on the powerful American Kennel Club, and its breeders, who were registering over 500,000 litters of puppies annually?

Why were the large respectable animal welfare organizations still making a distinction between puppy-millers and so-called responsible breeders. Can't we as intelligent people understand that when the lives of millions of innocent dogs and cats are lost each year to pet overpopulation, the term responsible breeder becomes an oxymoron?

Although we were asking these questions in the eighties and the nineties, as late as June 5, 2007, the Humane Society of the United States was still making a distinction between good breeders and bad breeders. On that date, the Lawton Constitution reported, from an Associated Press article, that Oklahoma is among the nation's worst states for puppy mill auctions, according to HSUS, who had completed an investigation.

Stephanie Shane, HSUS director of outreach, said in Missouri, breeders buy and sell dogs on a weekly basis in barns, and in Oklahoma and elsewhere the auctions happen openly, and sell at least 250 dogs on each occasion.

In spite of the horrors of pet breeding in that article, an Associated Press picture of puppy mill dogs in wire cages appeared, along with recommendations from the Humane Society of the United States on how to buy a dog—from a breeder!—"the humane way."

That drives me freakin' crazy! Oh, what the hell! It drives me fucking crazy. Why mince words? Why wasn't HSUS demanding statewide breeding laws from legislators that would tax breeding and provide much needed revenue for their coffers, and offset the negative financial impact of tax-supported animal shelter operations–and, most importantly end the nightmarish suffering of an endless number of voiceless dogs? And, even if HSUS was asking for legislation, as they sometimes have, how can you continue to advocate buying dogs from responsible breeders in the same breath you ask for legislation? The message is: "If you don't buy, they won't breed."

Why, we were asking, were animal advocates not insisting that local council members and city staff attend euthanasia sessions at local animal shelters? It is, after all, an integral function of city government with which they should acquaint themselves as they do with streets and highway departments, water treatment plants, etc. I once took the mayor of Lawton to view the god-awful scene of dead animals we had just euthanized.

Knowing full well of the feral cat problem in every community in the nation and cognizant of the fact that most farmers and dairymen refuse to neuter and spay barn cats, why are we not demanding that pet food manufacturers develop and place on the market affordable birth control pet food, especially in the cat food line?

Where were the billboards promoting the shame of breeding pets for profit?

Now that we'd finally started to ask questions, the one looming largest in our minds was: Why isn't pet overpopulation at the forefront of the Animal Rights Movement?

I took to the phone. Surely, I thought, I could find someone, somewhere, anywhere—far away from Oklahoma—perhaps in the metropolitan areas of Washington, D.C., or New York, that would understand my frustration, my anger, my pain about the senseless killing of dogs and cats for the last 150 years. I don't think I was being impatient or unreasonable. One hundred and fifty years?

I made calls to various organizations. No luck.

I made repeated calls to Ingrid Newkirk, founder of PETA. These people have funds. They have name recognition. They are bold and daring. They put pictures of naked women on billboards, for God's sake! Surely, if the PETA machine went into action, the ending of pet overpopulation would be a done deal.

I left my name. I left my number. Repeatedly. No luck.

Finally, one morning, at my wit's end, after participating in the euthanasia of several cats, in tears, and feeling I couldn't face any of this any longer, I phoned the PETA office again. This time I wasn't nice. I was put through to Ms. Newkirk.

Like a pleading child, I stated my case for the cause of pet overpopulation to this woman I understood to be a goddess in the struggle to liberate animals from pain, suffering and death. I explained to Ms. Newkirk that I realized pet overpopulation was not one of the more trendy issues of the movement, such as fur, tuna and whales.

After taking exception to my use of the word trendy, Ms. Newkirk did offer comforting words by telling me that pet overpopulation was being "talked about" in some of the large animal rights circles. And, finally, and sympathetically, she advised me to take B vitamins for my stress.

Somehow taking B vitamins wasn't the answer I was so desperately seeking. I wanted relief from this ache in my soul for the helpless, innocent lives I had just ended.

What is it, I thought, about society and even the Animal Rights Movement that shuns the tragic plight of "man's best friend?"

There is—there must be—I thought, some unwritten and unspoken conspiracy among certain groups, i.e. veterinarians, breeders, pet food companies—those who profit from a surplus of dogs and cats. But there couldn't be a conspiracy amongst our own, could there?

I frightened myself. What was wrong with me? What is it about me that keeps on believing that companion animals are as important as any aspect of the Animal Rights Movement?

I allowed those thoughts to taint my mind for only a fleeting moment. Then, as memories of untold numbers of beautiful, abandoned, emaciated animals, for whom I have grieved, jolted me back into the realm of sanity and reality, I realized, unequivocally, there is nothing wrong with me.

There is, however, something very wrong with a system, or a social movement, that views the slaughter of millions of pets each year, at taxpayer expense, as unworthy of serious consideration.

I called Linda, and other supporters, and we made the decision to continue a project we had discussed for months.

We would expand our local organization to a national organization with one focus and one focus only: to end pet overpopulation.

We would call it clearly and simply: The National Organization to End Pet Overpopulation.

NOPO.

CHAPTER 41

"Never doubt that a small group of thoughtful, committed citizens can change the world. In fact, it's the only thing that ever has."
— Margaret Mead

THE LETTER FROM the Internal Revenue Service was dated October 15, 1990. It gave us permission to change our name to The National Organization to End Pet Overpopulation, and advised us that the "changes indicated do not adversely affect your exempt status and the exemption letter issued to you continues in effect."

So what do we do now? A national organization out of Lawton, Oklahoma, seemed . . . well, it seemed almost laughable. But Walmart made it out of Bentonville, Arkansas, with a population of just over 40,000. Admittedly, our ambitions were probably somewhere outside the perimeters of reality.

My husband had set me to thinking sometime in early 1990 when he said to me, "You know, Deloris, it's just a shame you're working so hard in Lawton, and not in a larger city. No matter what you do here, it's still just Lawton; and it takes no more energy or money to fight the battles in a larger city than it does in this small town."

He was right! We were going to awaken a nation to the tragic consequences of pet overpopulation. No one else seemed to be doing it. It just didn't appear to be on the list of any of the large, wealthy organizations' priorities. But, by damned, we were going to do it!

Even the well-respected animal rights activist and writer Ed Duvin couldn't shake the animal sheltering establishment out of its complacency.

At about this same time, the now defunct Animals' Voice Magazine in California published two articles, "Benign Neglect" and "In the Name of Mercy," by Duvin. The articles accurately portrayed the animal sheltering establishment, which Duvin referred to as a "slumbering giant" uninspired to revolt against their daily routine killings.

I was ecstatic. His words eloquently paralleled my own thinking about the tragedy of pet overpopulation, and the neglect of even those among our own ranks to seriously address it.

Duvin pointed out the shameful non-existence of national shelter statistics. "Although shelters have existed in this country for well over a century, there is simply no reliable statistical base from which even the most basic information can be derived."

At that time, the number of animals killed in animal shelters had been set at 18 million annually. Currently, the no-kill movement wants us to believe it is only three or four million. One radical no-kill advocate, Nathan Winograd, insists that pet overpopulation doesn't exist at all, to which my newly made friend and animal advocate Beverly Perry responds, "I have pet overpopulation in my bedroom." This is someone who didn't realize what pet overpopulation was until she read this book.

No matter what website you visit, or who you speak to, everyone has a different number for animal shelter killings—simply because no one knows.

"How can we properly analyze where we have been, where we are at, where we are going, and how we're going to get there without reliable measurement?" Duvin had asked, all those years ago.

He emphasized that the public has "little or no understanding of the horrendous magnitude" of the tragedy of pet overpopulation.

"Compounding the problem," he said, "when the public is reached, the message they receive is "sanitized" with enough euphemisms to fill the Grand Canyon.

"Why isn't the unadulterated truth, stripped of any veneer, imaginatively and assertively brought to the public?

"What we should be doing is removing the killing from behind closed doors and informing the public about their role in the massive slaughter of our so-called closest companions."

Were we finally waking up to the realities and horrors of our insane method of animal control in this country?

Was someone finally admitting that, just possibly, humane societies and shelters have been on the wrong paths with the same old compromising attempts at solving the problem?

And, yes, finally someone was daring to trample—ever so lightly—on the sanctimony of purebred breeders.

Duvin wrote that pet breeding should be made to carry no less stigma than wearing fur, and blamed those who breed for any reason for their complicity in perpetuating the confinement and killing of precious beings.

Although I was encouraged by Duvin's article, my optimism, however, was guarded. Dr. Faulkner's earnest plea to veterinarians forty-nine years ago was circling in my brain. He had been unable to wake up or motivate his colleagues in this age-old pet overpopulation debacle.

Would Duvin be able to wake up the sheltering community?

Duvin and I shared phone conversations and letters. On April 1, 1991, he hand-penned a fairly lengthy letter to me discussing our mutual observations regarding the pet overpopulation issue. In an earlier letter, he had requested a copy of our no-chain ordinance, which I had provided.

"I'll be making good use of your no-chain ordinance," he wrote. "It's a model for others to emulate, and I agree that it also has an impact on overpopulation by discouraging irresponsible people from obtaining a pet.

I had sent him a copy of a study on pet overpopulation I had found from Minnesota. "You're right, Deloris, the Minnesota Legislative Report makes excellent reading, but the glaring omission of breeders leaves a gaping hole. I noticed the vets also took good care of themselves. So what else is new!"

He was complimentary of the goals of our new NOPO organization, and the literature and brochures we had produced.

In a letter dated November 8, 1991, he wrote: "I greatly admire your courage in taking this leap of faith, and I hope the response is tremendous. Thanks for being there, Deloris, and for bringing the ideals I wrote about in 'In the Name of Mercy' to life!"

But, alas, Duvin didn't wake up the sheltering community. He outraged them, along with many of the large national organizations.

The article was looked upon as a blame piece and it was unfair, thought many in the movement, to blame the sheltering establishment.

I had agreed with everything Duvin had observed and written about. But what has come out of those articles is the no-kill movement, which still falls short of being blameless. The Internet describes Duvin as "father of the no-kill movement."

If it is true that Duvin's articles spawned the no-kill movement, then I would point out that in "In the Name of Mercy" he describes the shelter experience for animals as a "kind of psychological trauma and terror that we find so abhorrent for caged laboratory animals but tolerate in our own facilities. Some are exposed to various forms of physical mishandling and abuse, and all suffer from the anguishing ordeal of being processed and warehoused in a foreign and frightening environment."

He admits that "euthanasia might be a relatively painless end to this journey of terror," but correctly points out that "each death represents an abject failure - not an act of mercy."

If Duvin's description of animals "being processed and warehoused" describes shelters who practice euthanasia, how does it exempt no-kill shelters, most of which cannot accept many animals brought to them—due to overcrowding?

CHAPTER 42

"If you want to get what you haven't gotten yet, then you have to do more than what you were doing before." — M. F. Moonzajer, Journalist

SINCE THIS NEW organization would consume even more of my time than was already being gobbled up by this cause, we sold *The Lawton Times* to John Dickerson, the managing editor. John and I would later work together for seven months writing the script of a 28-minute documentary/infomercial for television.

We started out first with direct mail. We found one of those companies who sell lists of labels with names of people known to donate to animal organizations. Those were the days when things were not as simple as the click of the mouse. Computers were not yet the world wide web we have become accustomed to. If you wanted to know something, you had to do a lot of digging around and making phone calls—on land lines, of all things!

We bought a permit for bulk mailing for non-profit organizations, and had envelope-stuffing parties where volunteers met and hand-folded letters and placed the sticky labels on the envelopes.

"We're mad as hell and we're not taking it anymore." Well, we didn't actually write those words in our first direct mail solicitation, but that was the gist of the message. We began our letter thusly: "It makes no sense! And we at The National Organization to End Pet Overpopulation (NOPO) are angry! We've seen enough! We're waging a war!"

"We're angry because year after year an estimated 18,000,000 of this nation's pets—like your own Spot or Lady or Mitzie—are herded into death rooms and killed at animal shelters across the country."

We said we were angry about abandoned pets on highways and the billions of American tax dollars spent to collect, shelter and kill the nation's pets.

"Recently, the animal movement has succeeded in many worthwhile endeavors—from crippling the fur industry to convincing major cosmetic companies to end animal testing," we wrote.

We told readers pet overpopulation is a solvable problem that hasn't been given the attention, commitment, and determination it so desperately deserves.

"Your donation won't be divided into a number of various animal projects," we promised. It will be used for one cause and one cause only: To wage war on pet overpopulation."

We included pictures of a euthanasia room full of animals, a kitten and a dog in cages, and a photo of the pitiful emaciated greyhounds, which was still so strongly embedded in our minds.

Our triple-fold color brochure pictured a flatbed trailer loaded with beautiful, once-healthy, dead dogs and cats headed for the Lawton landfill.

We had no qualms whatsoever about exposing the horrors of pet overpopulation to an uninformed nation. It was about time!

We had ordered a video, wherein a beautiful Irish Setter, whose name was Jo Jo, was euthanized for television viewing. We had used it locally to assist us in promoting breeding laws. It can be viewed on our website today.

We were pleasantly surprised at the response to our correspondence. An assistant professor at North Adams State College in Massachusetts was understandably cautious. "I am very sympathetic with pets," she said, "and I want to help. I hope you will understand my caution," she wrote. "If you are as legitimate as your literature would lead me to believe, you have 100% of my support."

Other letters broke our hearts. One lady from Cedar Creek, Texas, wrote: "I would be more than happy to help, but I am on disability, and can barely make it myself." The woman explained that she lives in the country and has dogs that were dropped off near her home. "I could not see them starve or to be hit with a car. I took them in, but if I cannot find help soon, I will have to be one of the countless hundreds who take dogs to the Humane society to be distroyed (sic)."

Whether or not we were able to help this woman, I can't recall. I hope so. On the back of her letter, I have the name of a veterinarian in her area, prices for surgery, the woman's sister's name, the ages of the dogs, and questions I had asked someone about the dogs.

A woman in Hendersonville, North Carolina, sent a donation of $20.00, explaining it was "unfortunately" all she could give at the time. She also had a pet overpopulation problem of her own. "We had a total of nine (9) stray cats appear at our home this spring." She told us she gave them to a dairy farmer without having them neutered and spayed. She had contacted her local humane society for help, but they had no room.

She continued to write that another mother cat and two kittens arrived, which she kept and built a screened-in porch onto her house for their protection.

"My sister and I took on a weekend job to earn the money to have these cats neutered, have their vaccinations, buy cat food, and be able to provide veterinary care when needed," she wrote.

She spoke of another cat she named Phantom, who arrived and for whom she provided a wooden box on her front porch. She caught Phantom in a trap, had her spayed, and released her. "She disappeared about two weeks ago," the woman lamented. The burden is heavy with me that she, too, never knew the comfort of a real home. Unless she's found it now!

"We have had two or three years' worth of trying to find homes for about two dozen cats and one dog," she continued. And it's close to the most heart-rending experience I've ever had—surpassing in burden even the loss of family members. At least I know THEY are OK!"

She explained she wanted to keep up with the progress of our organization. "The only solution I see to this horrible problem is to somehow control reproduction. Good luck to you—and us!" Those letters were typical of the stories we heard from bewildered rescuers across America.

IN 1992, WE FORMED what we called the NOPO 2000 Task Force. Our goal was to end pet overpopulation by the year 2000. We would ask Americans to join with us by making the following commitment: Always have their own pets neutered and spayed, never allowing them to have even one litter; Always adopt from animal shelters rather than buying from pet shops or breeders. The NOPO motto has always been:"If you don't buy, they won't breed." And, finally, we would ask America to support laws that restrict and tax all pet breeding.

After seven months of script-writing, with the help of John Dickerson, we produced a twenty-eight minute, high quality, made-for-television video entitled NOPO 2000. This was in 1991.

We were amazed at the number of prominent people in Lawton and surrounding areas who agreed to appear in the video. John, who had a degree in broadcast journalism, served as the announcer in the film. Local KSWO Channel 7 TV anchor woman, Tamara Pratt, agreed to host the show. In a year or so, she moved on to a larger television market in Oklahoma City.

From the steps of the Oklahoma State Capitol, State Senator Roy "Butch" Hooper talked about the need for legislation controlling pet breeding; local Judge Kenny Harris spoke about the validity of our plan to tackle pet overpopulation nationwide; former Councilman and current County Commissioner Frank Walker spoke about Oklahoma puppy mills and the need for breeding laws.

Kathy McKee, a spokesperson for Americans Against Puppy Mills, drove all the way from Kansas City to do a ninety-second spot about the horrors of puppy mills in her state.

Jan Pierce from Texas told of her heartbreaking nightmares from her years of shelter work. Jan began having dreams about euthanizing dogs and cats. As a teacher, she also began to dream of euthanizing her classroom children. Then in one horrible nightmare, Jan was being forced to euthanize her own children. At that point, she gave up shelter work.

Jerry Owens, Lawton's shelter supervisor of the month, at that time, talked about the shame of killing animals, and the need for heavily-enforced breeding laws; and a local woman spoke of the hardships she had endured, including having to borrow money to send her daughter to college, from caring for too many strays.

A professional televison personality from Oklahoma City plead with viewers to join our Task Force by sending a donation of $25 and agreeing to the commitment to end overpopulation by the year 2000. We, in turn, offered a donor the choice of a NOPO 2000 Task Force member tee shirt or a coffee mug emblazoned with the NOPO 2000 Task Force logo.

We purchased, mostly, late night spots which were less expensive, but, on some occasions we were able to get the video on prime time. Because of lack of funds, we set up our own 1-800 number, and three or four of us would man the phones when the video was on the air.

Again, we were amazed at the response. Not so much at the volume of the calls, or certainly not because we were raking in money, but because so many viewers were suffering from the same problems we had experienced for so many years.

One woman wrote: "All I can say is THANK YOU! My husband and I have taken in so many homeless animals that it is impossible to take anymore."

On June 28, 1992, a lady from Texas wrote: "Friday night, I stayed up to watch Love Connection on Channel 7. Instead I was pleasantly surprised to see your ad. I had never before heard of your organization, which shares my views and wishes to a T."

She said she found it a mystery why city governments don't tap a source of revenue readily available, by requiring tags on all animals with minimal costs for those spayed and neutered, and high for "breedable" animals.

A young Texas beauty contestant wrote: "This is such a huge problem and it seems almost no one is interested in diminishing it."

She explained that she had formerly been Miss Wichita Falls and was now Miss Plano, which is a suburb of Dallas. "This will be my second year to compete in the Miss Texas Scholarship Pageant." She was so interested in what NOPO stood for, she offered to be a national spokesperson if she were to win the Miss America title.

She ended her letter with: "You don't know how excited I am that NOPO exists."

Not everyone was excited about NOPO. We got calls attempting to jam the phone lines, which obviously were from breeders. A San Diego, California, humane organization must have felt we were infringing on their territory when it aired in that area. They asked us for our Form 990, which we promptly produced.

But perhaps the most threatened of anyone was the American Kennel Club. It didn't take long for the New York City organization to get wind of this televison show. They actually ran ads in local newspapers warning of "animal rights extremists."

One such ad was entitled: "Information Bulletin from the American Kennel Club. BE INFORMED.

"The American Kennel Club wants to make you aware that there are people in this country who have launched a well-organized campaign to take away your rights to breed and own pure-bred dogs. These people are members of those extreme animal rights groups that think no one should "own" a companion animal.

"There is a substantial difference between animal rights and animal welfare. Animal rights extremists are advocating the end of pure-bred dogs. Animal welfare asks that we provide proper care and love for the entire life of our dogs. Remember that not all animal rights people are extremists. The common ground is that no one wants to see dogs suffer. The American Kennel Club supports the best premises of animal welfare and is opposed to any groups trying to take away your right to be responsible breeders and owners. The AKC has many new and exciting programs addressing these issues, but we need the support and cooperation of the entire fancy to have maximum impact.

"Please take the time to learn the hidden agendas of any organization when you donate time or money. Some of the very organizations that are opposed to companion animal ownership receive daily donations from dog fanciers. Also, learn about the laws that affect dog ownership where you live. Make certain your dogs are secure at all times, especially during dog shows. And perhaps most important, join your local dog federation or organize one if one does not exist in your area.

"The American Kennel Club can help you become informed. For more information about AKC positions on current canine issues, breeding bans, legislation, or responsible breeding, write to us." The ad was tagged The American

Kennel Club, Communications Division, 51 Madison Avenue, New York, New York 10010—a long distance from the dog farms in the boondocks of the State of Oklahoma.

It was hard to know where to start to address the bull shit that was in that ad. I especially loved the warning to breeders about keeping their dogs "secure at all times, especially during dog shows."

Oh yeah! Just what we needed. Did we not have enough dogs to deal with every day of our lives? Did they actually think we needed to go to an AKC show and steal us a few more dogs?

I don't think so!

We countered the AKC's untruths about our organization with our own ad. It was entitled: "Information Bulletin From the National Organization To End Pet Overpopulation. Be Informed."

"The National Organization to End Pet Overpopulation wants to make you aware that there are people in this country whose hearts are breaking because millions of excess pets are being bred and must be killed each year. Many of these are the same people whose lives are overwhelmed by trying to care for too many pets; or they are the same people who work in shelters and must kill innocent, beautiful pets day after day, month after month, year after year—pets that are both mixed breeds and purebreds. And they are ordinary taxpayers who are sick of knowing their tax dollars are spent to impound and kill pets purely because there are too many bred.

"These are the same people who are often labeled radical by those who continually fight against any form of controls or limits on pet breeding which causes animals to be killed by the millions. These people are obviously motivated by financial gain rather than a genuine desire to end pet overpopulation.

"Please take the time to learn things that you should know: For instance, the American Kennel Club registered 567,763 litters (yes, that's litters) of puppies in 1991 at $15 per litter. They registered 1,379,544 individual dogs at $7 per single dog. This amounts to millions of dollars in registration fees for the American Kennel Club. Is it any wonder they are so adamantly opposed to any controls over breeding? Is it possible that the AKC doesn't even have the best interests of its breeders at heart considering the fact that the availability of too many pets keeps their sale value lower?

"The National Organization to End Pet Overpopulation is motivated only by our concern for abandoned and dying pets and what it means in human and animal suffering and in tax dollars that are necessary to deal with the surpluses. What motivates the AKC and pet breeders? The answer is obvious."

It was almost comical to see that our little organization, who existed on a day-to-day shoestring budget, had threatened the New York City giant.

It would not be the last time, however, that we would hear from the powerful American Kennel Club here in Lawton, or in the State of Oklahoma.

AS FOR NOPO, we were on our way. I was visualizing a line of clothing with the NOPO message: "If you don't buy, they won't breed." I had four grandsons who were skateboarders; and I was envisioning the NOPO name alongside such familiar board clothing lines, at that time, as Alien Workshop, Chocolate, Girl, and Quicksilver. I wanted to educate America's youth about pet overpopulation.

We visualized NOPO low-cost neuter/spay clinics sitting alongside Walmart, McDonald's, Target, and other chains—on street corners across the nation.

Yes, The National Organization to End Pet Overpopulation in Lawton, Oklahoma, who had successfully intimidated the American Kennel Club in New York City, was on its way to changing the world.

But a funny thing happened on the way to changing the world!

CHAPTER 43

"The creatures outside looked from pig to man, and from man to pig, and from pig to man again; but already it was impossible to say which was which." — George Orwell, *Animal Farm*

"NOW LET ME see if I have this straight," mused the puzzled emergency room doctor, as he looked at the broken skin on my right arm. "You work at the humane society, and you've been bitten by a human?"

Actually, I had. I had been bitten by a human. In this intriguing world of animal welfare that I had gotten myself into, I was now one for one. One bite by a dog, a tiny Chihuahua, and one bite by a human, a grown adult woman.

The young woman, who had left her teeth marks on my arm, had recently been hired to work at the clinic. She had taken a fancy to a stray puppy, and had asked for permission to take it home overnight. Initially, seeing no harm in her request, we allowed her to take the small dog home. She was to return it to the clinic the next morning, a Saturday, but she didn't show up with the little dog.

Linda and I were concerned about the fact that she had not done as she had promised. We decided to go to her residence and bring the puppy back to the clinic.

We arrived at the woman's duplex, knocked on the door and she, reluctantly, released the puppy to us without much fanfare.

No sooner had we returned the puppy to the clinic and were settling him into his kennel, when we realized we had been followed by the woman, who came inside the building, and proceeded to grab up the dog, and head for the front door. Linda immediately picked up the phone, which was on the desk, near the front door, to call the police and report an attempted theft of a dog. As the girl attempted to run out the door, I put up my right arm in front of her in an effort to stop her. She bent over and bit my arm hard enough for me to yell at Linda for help.

"Linda," I yelped, "help me, she's biting me."

Not knowing what else to do, and later admitting that this may not have been one of her finer moments, Linda smacked the woman on the head with the phone receiver to get her attention.

This young woman was incorrigible. Undaunted by the strike on her head, she continued to run out of the building, still clinging to the dog. As Linda went after her, she started to hit at Linda, who was now becoming frightened of her. I don't know if there is such an affliction as puppy obsession, but if so, this woman had a severe case of it.

By now, two police officers had arrived. The woman immediately headed over to talk to them with the puppy still clenched in her arms.

Linda also approached the police. "I'm the one who called you." she said. "Shouldn't you be talking to me first?"

I had followed Linda outside. We were both ordered, however, by one of the officers, "to get back inside the building."

Amazingly, the two police officers were actually arguing in favor of the girl who was attempting to steal the puppy. They insisted we had no proof the dog belonged to us.

"Why do you think we called you," Linda snapped. "To report that we were stealing her puppy?" Finally, after what seemed like hours of combative rhetoric back and forth, I remembered something that might make the police believe us.

"If you think this girl owns this puppy," I said, "then ask her to show you her adoption papers. I'll bet she can't do that," I chided. I showed the officers our adoption forms.

"If she has legally adopted this puppy from us, she will have this paperwork as well as vaccination records. Ask her to show you those." I requested.

I was proud of myself. I felt like a lawyer in a courtroom, a Perry Mason type, who had just revealed a new surprising piece of evidence that would break the case wide open, and we would walk out of the parking lot courtroom as joyous victors.

Sure enough, my hunch worked. When the woman could not produce the adoption papers, the police, obviously feeling they had no other choice, instructed the would-be puppy thief to give us back our puppy.

The police and the woman left the clinic. Linda and I were left standing in the parking lot, clutching the puppy, looking at each other in bewilderment, and thinking: "What the hell just happened here?"

We weren't, however, taking any chances with this crazy woman. Another employee took the dog home overnight, and eventually adopted it herself.

Linda took one look at my arm and talked me into going to the emergency room.

IF ONLY THE puppy incident had been fresher in my mind, I might never have placed a call to the Lawton police station on that fateful Saturday night in July 1992.

CHAPTER 44

"The nail that sticks out farthest gets hammered the hardest." — Patrick Jones, *Nailed*

KELLYE DUBBER, A humane society volunteer, and I had been out on a Saturday night, attempting to trap a dog I had been feeding for months, or maybe even a year.

"You probably need to try to get that dog," my husband had said to me a day or so earlier. "She looks like she's been hit by a car. She's limping pretty bad."

The dog in question looked to be a black lab mix. It was impossible to get within fifty feet of her. She hung out in a vacant field on East Gore Boulevard, a well-traveled Lawton street. She lived life on her own terms, and was not to be caught.

I had probably been unable to trap her because, unbeknown to me, she was being fed by other people, and was never hungry enough to venture into the unknown environment of a wire trap.

The sports bar and restaurant right across the street most likely had fed her occasionally; and I would find out, when she finally died, still running as a stray, that she was also being fed by a kind, middle-aged man I had never met. He must have known I, too, was feeding the dog because he came to the clinic to let me know that she was dead; and that he had buried her body. I will never know what took her life. It, hopefully, was natural causes from old age.

This dog was strange. I had purchased her a dog house with bedding, and set it in the field where she was usually seen, however, she was all over the place—up and down East Gore Boulevard.

My husband's dealership was on Gore and when we drove into town, we would see the dog on a daily basis.

As might be expected, someone stole the dog house. I asked Rain's Maytag, a local appliance store whose owner is a strong animal advocate, for a large washing machine box. I then had a carpenter make a smaller wooden, insulated dog house and we slid it right inside the washing machine box. The property on which I needed to place the box was tribal land, and I received permission to sit this dog house, camouflaged as a simple piece of trash, to the back of the field. No one bothered to mess with it again.

I don't believe, however, that this strange dog ever used that shelter. I would drive by, and it would be pouring rain, or snowing, and there this dog would be — lying down, right out in the middle of that field, and seeming to be enjoying it.

KELLYE AND I were having no luck at all with this streetwise canine. I wasn't surprised. It wasn't the first time she had outsmarted us. It was almost ten o'clock when I called my husband to tell him we hadn't been able to get the dog; and that we were going to give it a little more time, as we had seen her cross the street and head back to where we had set the trap.

By this time, our kids were all grown, and Dan had gotten accustomed to spending time at home alone while I was out on animal missions. Of course, that's not to say he was always happy about it and that there weren't arguments. When he became frustrated with it all, he would say, "Animals, animals, animals. That's all our life is about. Animals!" Overall, he had the patience of Job, and without his generous support, my work with animals would have not been possible.

By the time I finished speaking to Dan, Kellye and I were turning into the one-way, two-lane drive at Taco Mayo. A police unit, however, was parked in an angled position blocking the entrance. The officer had pulled over a pick up, and the driver had parked in one of the marked parking spaces. I noticed that if the officer would just move her unit a couple of feet, traffic coming into Taco Mayo could either park or head to the drive-thru.

I calmly stepped out of the pickup, and politely spoke to the officer.

"Ma'am," I said. "Could you please move your vehicle? You're blocking the drive."

I genuinely thought this officer should not be blocking a business drive because of an experience I'd had a few years before. Unthinking, I had illegally made a right-hand turn, on a red light, at one of the very few intersections in Lawton where it is not legal to do so. An officer had motioned me to pull over, and I had driven into the parking lot of the nearby Chevrolet dealership.

Almost immediately, after stopping our vehicles, the manager of the dealership came outside and demanded we move our cars, inasmuch as we were on private property. The police officer directed me to move my car, and he followed suit.

In this case, the officer whose vehicle was blocking traffic on private property, was a woman officer who I would later learn was Diane Jones. She told me she was making an arrest.

"Okay. That's reasonable," I said to Kellye, as I stepped back into the pickup. Kellye and I sat chatting for about twenty minutes. We watched, more or less intrigued, as the officer directed an elderly woman to walk a straight line, touch her nose, and perform other tasks of a field sobriety test. Finally, the officer handcuffed the woman and placed her in the back seat of the police vehicle.

Kellye and I said, almost simultaneously, "Well, finally. Maybe now she'll move her car." That didn't happen. Instead the officer opened the door on the driver's side of her vehicle and took out what looked to be a clipboard, and proceeded to mosey around the arrested lady's truck, looking at the tires, just doing what appeared to be busy work.

Frustrated, I again stepped out of my pickup and asked her to please move her car. She completely ignored me.

What was interesting was that Dan and I owned this property. We had it leased to the owners of Taco Mayo. I had never planned to mention any of this to this woman, but I was remembering the incident at the Chevrolet dealership; and this just didn't seem right. After twenty minutes, I went inside to determine if the owners were there, and see what they thought about this blockage of the entry to their restaurant on a Saturday night.

While we were parked, other cars had attempted to enter the drive.

"This is just not safe," said one woman, as she backed out of the drive with a carload of children. When I learned the owners of the restaurant were not there, I went back to the truck. Once again, I asked the officer to move her vehicle. Again, she completely ignored me. I then told her we owned the property, thinking this might bear some weight with her. Nothing. No response.

I was getting angry. I should have just left. And I did. But not before I called the police station.

"This is Mrs. Delluomo," I said. There's a police unit number 156 at Taco Mayo out on East Gore that's blocking a business drive, and I'm wondering if she should be able to do that?"

Notice that I said, "This is Mrs. Delluomo." Would anyone in their right mind give their name over the phone if they believed, for a moment, they were doing anything wrong, or they would wind up in jail as a result of that call?

I was told the officer could indeed do what she was doing if she was making an arrest. "No," I explained. "She's already made her arrest. The arrested woman is in her car."

The person on the phone at the police department told me to hold on. I could tell he was calling Officer Jones, as we could see her talking on her radio.

"She can't move that vehicle," explained the voice on the phone. "It's being impounded. Isn't there another exit out there?"

"No," I said. "You don't understand. It is not the vehicle belonging to the lady being arrested. It's the police vehicle that's blocking the drive."

This was ridiculous. It was no longer worth the trouble. I finally said, "Oh, just forget it. She's not going to move her vehicle. She's just showing us her authority. She's had plenty of time to do it; she's just not going to do it."

"She's not showing her authority; she's doing her job," said the increasingly angry voice on the other end of the line.

"No. She's already done her job, and it's very obvious what she's doing now. But just forget it," I said for a second time. "You're the police and I guess you can do whatever you want." I hung up the phone.

Kellye and I backed out into traffic on Gore Boulevard; and that was the end of that—or so we thought.

I called Dan when we were leaving the restaurant, still with no food or drink, and told him of the incident. I told him he might just drive down by Taco Mayo, if he didn't have anything better to do, and look at how this police unit was blocking the drive; and that if she only moved her vehicle a couple of feet, cars could get by her unit. I told him we were going to go pick up the dog trap and I would be heading home.

I would, however, not make it home for hours.

As Kellye and I drove back to the west to check our trap, we noticed a police "Supervisor" unit heading east on the opposite side of the center median.

"Oh, look," Kellye beamed. "There's a police supervisor. I guess he's going to check things out after all."

Kellye's optimism was short-lived. That was not what the supervisor was doing. He had left his post at the police station, on a Saturday night, and put out an all points bulletin to stop my truck—because he was determined to check me out!

Lt. Michael Burch was one of the officers who had been summoned by the radio transmission. He knew our family. He radioed Lt. Mathis to ask if he should go out and talk to me.

"No, I'll take care of her," replied Mathis.

IT SEEMED LT. Mathis was desperately searching for a reason to arrest me. He had asked for a rundown on my driver's license to check for warrants, and that hadn't panned out for him. He had called the officer at Taco Mayo to see if she had "enough" to arrest me for interference, and she was obviously sketchy on that. What was he to do?

Officer Burch was on the passenger side of the truck speaking to Kellye, who was on the phone placing a call to Dan.

"You need to put the phone down," the officer ordered Kelly, but not before she had finished telling Dan, in a panic, that he needed to "come down here. They are trying to arrest us."

At some point, in the midst of this insane event that was taking place in the middle of a gravel parking lot, I had stepped back into my husband's truck and rested my hands on the steering wheel.

By this time, I was pleading with Officer Mathis to just let us go; that we had done nothing wrong; and that we needed to check our dog trap.

"Please, can we just go now?" I begged.

"You're not going anywhere," said Officer Mathis.

I have admitted in a previous chapter that I am a flawed person and that patience is not one of my redeeming traits. Lt. Mathis had nothing with which to hold us, yet he would not let us go.

"You're an asshole," I said, looking straight into the face of this police officer who wanted nothing more than to see me in jail; and I had given him just what he was looking for.

"That's it! You're under arrest!" said officer Mathis as he grabbed onto my wrists and dragged me from the pickup.

Lt. Mathis was manhandling me in a way that was painful. He grabbed me by my upper left arm and jerked me out of the truck. He then took hold of my wrist and twisted it to get it behind me in order to handcuff me. I was spinning around attempting to move myself in the direction of the twist of my arm because he was seriously hurting me. I knew he wanted to hurt me. By the time he handcuffed me, I was almost on my knees.

At about the exact time Officer Mathis was handcuffing me, my husband had driven onto the crime scene.

Anyone who knew my husband knew him to be a gentle, laid back human being. He got out of his car with his hands in the pockets of his jeans, and was attempting to assess what was happening. When he heard me screaming that Mathis was hurting me, he headed in my direction, only to be jumped on by the other three officers.

In the midst of all this, Kellye, too, had been arrested. As we were being walked, handcuffed, to the patrol car, we walked past Dan who was struggling to get free from the officers to come to my aid. I actually was afraid for all of us.

"Please, Dan," I said. "Don't fight with them. We'll get lawyers for this."

"I'm not doing anything." he said. "They're all over me."

How did a simple effort to rescue a black stray dog ever turn into such a disastrous, life-changing event?

CHAPTER 45

"The hallmark of courage in our age of conformity is the capacity to stand on one's own convictions–not obstinately or defiantly (these are gestures of defensiveness, not courage) nor as a gesture of retaliation, but simply because these are what one believes." — Rollo May, Psychologist, Author, 1909-1994

GETTING THE STRAY black dog should have been a job for animal control. Knowing what I knew about them, however, they were the last people I would have called for help.

If they had tried to get the dog, I was thankful it was too smart for them. A beautiful stray cocker spaniel, running loose in a section of Lawton called "Old Town" had not been so lucky. Neither had a stray Sharpei.

On the day of July 25, 1992, the same day of the arrest, the Daily Oklahoman carried an article, written by Mark A. Hutchison, entitled: "Humane Society Influencing Case Attorney Says, Lawton Upholds Terminations."

"A Lawton attorney representing three animal control officers under fire for their roles in the deaths of two dogs says he believes city officials are being unfairly influenced by the humane society," wrote Hutchison.

"Art Mata said city manager Bob Hopkins' recent decision to veto a personnel board's recommendation that two of the officers be given their jobs back is unjustified. "He says he'll appeal the decision in district court.

"Animal control officers Vickie Payne, John McCall Jr. and Rudolph Lopez have come under scrutiny within the last few weeks after the three were fired last month," the article stated.

On February 5, 1992, two officers had been in pursuit of a cocker spaniel who had run into a detached garage with its door partially open.

Attorney Mata said the officers had "unsuccessfully attempted to notify the residence owner, but did not enter the garage for fear of breaking the law," according to the article.

The officers pushed down the garage door with the cocker spaniel trapped inside—and simply never went back.

Relatives of the elderly man, who owned the home, found the remains of the dog on May 28, 1992, after the man's death.

On June 5, 1992, the Lawton Constitution reported that a volunteer who was working with the animal control officers during a February 5 sweep of stray dogs reported the incident to the Humane Society of Comanche County.

"After the dog's remains were found, society officials demanded an investigation by the city," the article stated.

"Payne and McCall are accused of not following proper procedures when they euthanized a stray Sharpei dog on May 5," Hutchison also reported in the Daily Oklahoman article.

"The personnel board overturned the firings and instead approved unpaid suspensions for the three officers. Hopkins on Thursday vetoed the board's decision concerning Payne and McCall, and reaffirmed their termination.

"In a letter to board members, Hopkins said in part 'I believe that the board did not fully appreciate the seriousness of the offenses committed by Ms. Payne and Mr. McCall.' Hopkins upheld the board's decision concerning Lopez."

Hutchison quoted from a letter I had written to Payne informing her I was "sickened" over the death of the Sharpei because "we still have officers such as yourself who are more concerned with the thrill of the kill than they are in rescuing an abandoned, frightened and emaciated animal in a civilized or humane manner." Also in the letter, copies of which were given to city officials, I had promised if the inhumane practices didn't cease "I assure you the Humane Society will lead a citizen campaign to see that they do." The article quoted Hopkins as saying that "The letter alone had no influence."

There is no doubt the firing of the animal control officers cinched my status as a well-known, long-time Lawton trouble maker—as far as Lt. Mathis was concerned.

CHAPTER 46

"I have as much authority as the Pope. I just do not have as many people who believe it." — George Carlin, comedian

THE DOCUMENTS FROM that arrest and the trials that resulted over a period of the next few years could fill its own book; the arrest, however, is not the focus of this book. It does, however, go to show just how much trouble you can get into when you position yourself squarely in the middle of the animal welfare cause in this country—and fight hard for your beliefs.

IN TWO DIFFERENT trials, my husband and I were found "not guilty" of anything. Our lawyer then advised us to sue the City of Lawton for violation of our civil rights. That was not something we particularly wanted to do. All we ever wanted was an apology from the police or the city, and it would all have been forgotten. But that apology never came.

My husband was heartbroken about this incident—more so than I. In every testimony he gave in three different trials, he cried on the witness stand. His dealership was only a couple of blocks away from the police station. Two of the homicide detectives were friends with my son, and had come to the dealership for coffee, almost on a daily basis. The dealership had loaned automobiles to the police for undercover detective work, and Dan had donated to the Fraternal Order of Police. He felt betrayed.

I was the one, however, who probably had betrayed him. There was no doubt he had suffered that indignity with the police due to my animal advocacy—and the loud voice that went along with it.

OUR LAWSUIT AGAINST the city took place in Federal court. We were painted by the lawyers for the police as a wealthy family who believed we could do anything we wanted to do and get by with it.

The jurors came from all over the state, mostly from small rural communities, some clad in overalls, and I think they actually were convinced that we, especially me, were spoiled people—who didn't give the men in blue their due respect.

We, mistakenly, actually dressed the part for court. We purchased new suits especially for the trial, and dressed in them every day for weeks, believing that was what we were supposed to do, even though that didn't represent the way we lived our daily lives.

Dan was probably one of the only Nissan dealers in the United States who went to work every day in jeans and tennis shoes. He pretty much stayed in the background; never did his own TV ads; was not in sales. He quietly oversaw the daily operations of the business from a comfortable distance. I think the fact that he dressed so casually endeared him to his customers and friends.

Dan was known for his great sense of humor. He loved to tell the story about the salesman who drove up to the front door as he was standing in the middle of the showroom floor. He knew the salesman had come there to see him.

"Can I help you," he said, as the man walked straight past him. The stranger took a look at Dan in his casual attire.

"I don't think so," he said.

Dan stood in the same spot and quietly watched the suit-clad salesman make the rounds to the parts department, then to the service department, then to the office. Finally, the salesman returned to the spot where Dan was standing.

"I guess you're the person I need to see after all," he admitted.

Because I worked on a daily basis with animals, I, too, dressed in jeans more than any other attire. People who knew us knew we were not elitist people who disrespected the police. We didn't even attempt to run in socially prominent circles. We simply marched to our own drummer.

In his testimony, Mathis insisted our lawyer was trying to depict the police as violent officers "beating up on this lady and her husband similar to the Rodney King case, when indeed it's been dubbed—or she's been dubbed as the Zsa Zsa Gabor of Lawton," he told jurors.

"You're absolutely wrong, Mr. Mathis. You're a ruthless, corrupt police officer is what you are, absolutely," John Zelbst, our lawyer, said to Lt. Mathis, in a raised voice so familiar to courtroom drama.

"You've been fired. You've been suspended," Zelbst ranted, before the judge put an end to the combative dialogue.

Mathis admitted that his perception of us was that because of our bank account we could act differently than regular people.

"Tell me what you know about Mr. and Mrs. Delluomo's bank account?" Zelbst asked.

"I know they give a great deal of money to public officials in this community," Mathis said.

"How much is a great deal of money?" Zelbst quizzed.

"I would say several hundred to thousands of dollars," Mathis answered.

"What you're trying to say is because that they work hard and they have a business here, that they don't have to comply with the law, is that what you're saying?" Zelbst asked.

"There's a lot of underlying political things that go on behind the scene on this case, a lot, and you know more, Mr. Zelbst," Mathis said.

"I don't know what you're talking about, but I'm asking the question here, Mr. Mathis, are you saying that because they're successful with the business, that they don't have to follow the law?" Zelbst asked.

"I'm saying money talks," Mathis said.

Where Lt. Mathis got all his erroneous information I have no idea. This great wealth of ours that was being bantered about by the police and their defense attorneys was a myth. Yes, my husband worked hard and we lived a fairly comfortable life. We also recognized that we were blessed and we did our best to return some of our good fortune to the community—and my work in animal welfare was a part of that.

I would guess the underlying political "things" of which Lt. Mathis spoke had more to do with the animal cause, and the firing of the two animal control officers just a couple of days before the arrest, than it had to do with anything else. Admittedly, I did support the firing of the animal control officers and I urged the city manager to uphold his decision. An innocent, frightened cocker spaniel starved to death due to their indifference and lack of compassion. Why should they ever have been allowed to handle another animal for the City of Lawton and be paid to do so?

Hopkins had obviously agreed with me, thus his statement to the media about the "seriousness of the offenses committed by Ms. Payne and Mr. McCall."

If we donated to a political campaign, it was always a modest amount. We did, indeed, contribute to candidates who we believed would support animal causes in our community and state.

WE LOST OUR lawsuit against the city. I don't think my husband ever got over the miscarriage of justice we felt we experienced. It was never about the money. It was about justice.

Dan was always able, however, to keep his sense of humor, for which he was so well known. He considered purchasing a billboard with a message asking the question: "If you're under attack by the LPD, do you still call 911?"

DAN LOST INTEREST in the dealership after this unfortunate encounter with the police. He was getting tired. We both were getting tired. It would only be a short time before we would sell the business and take our leave for a place in the sun, leaving behind the Animal Birth Control Clinic, the humane society, Linda—and the entire heartbreaking world of animal welfare.

CHAPTER 47

"When the Man waked up he said, 'What is Wild Dog doing here?' And the woman said, 'His name is not Wild Dog any more, but the First Friend, because he will be our friend for always and always and always." — Rudyard Kipling

"SHE USED TO be beautiful; now she was just hungry and thirsty and tired and scared. You may know the dog I'm talking about. She's that German shepherd you saw trying to cross Highway 101. Or she's that beagle pup with six puppies of her own, living in the basement of a deserted house. Or she's that golden retriever that nobody wants anymore.

"He's never really known a happy moment in his whole life. No one's ever cared for him properly or loved him enough. You know the one I mean. He's the dog who's tied up in the back yard day and night. The one nobody feeds until the neighbors complain. Or he's the cat we read about in the newspapers. The one who was horribly beaten, or maybe brutally tormented. Or he's the dog who'll spend his life in a research laboratory. The one who lives in a small cage and "smokes" cigarettes all day long.

"They are exquisite. Why shouldn't they be! What could be more perfect than a box full of kittens! You know the ones I mean. The ones that were left on the steps of the police station one dark night. Or the ones that were stuffed into a garbage can and left to die. Or the ones that were dumped along the side of the road and left to fend for themselves.

"Some people don't see the connection between pet overpopulation and animal neglect, abuse and abandonment. They don't understand that when their cat has kittens, many other animals will suffer. But as long as cats and dogs are plentiful, they will be neglected, abused and discarded. There aren't enough good homes for all the animals who need them, so many animals end up in bad homes, or end up on the streets, or end up in research laboratories or end up in animal shelters.

"While you may think that the birth of six puppies or kittens is a celebration of life, we can tell you that every animal that is born in this country, whether mixed breed or purebred, planned or accidental, only reduces the chances that every cat or kitten, dog or puppy will find a good home. And if anything is discouraging about the field of animal welfare, it is the knowledge that people who care about their pets fail to see this connection. In doing so, they help to create a situation that is impossible for us to fix.

"You may not see the connection between the six St. Bernard puppies you just sold (to 'good homes'), and the fact that today we must destroy six dogs in our shelter alone. But that connection is real, and if you allow your pet to breed, you, too, have made a contribution to the problem of pet overpopulation.

"Many people think that purebred animals are not victims in this chain of animal mistreatment, but even expensive purebred animals cannot escape this cruel system. You may be surprised to know that purebred animals not only end up in animal shelters, they die there, too. They come in as strays, they come in as animal abuse cases, they're turned in by their owners because they've gotten too big or they chew up the furniture. A beautiful Irish setter, a charming Cairn terrier, an engaging Abyssinian: These, too, are part of the sad statistics. Nowadays even purebred animals are often treated like 'a dime a dozen.'

"We can also tell you that many 'mutts' are clearly halfbreeds. To regard all mixed-breed animals as the 'Heinz 57 Variety' is a mistake. The fact is, purebred animals produce many of our mixed-breed mutts. So when we get in a half German shepherd/half golden retriever or a half Manx/half Siamese, we know that somewhere there are purebred animals that are not being cared for properly. When it comes to pet overpopulation, purebred animals are not only beautiful victims, they are often prolific ones, too, and their days as the pampered members of animal society are over.

"Let's say that you do find good homes for a batch of six kittens. If your 'good homes' are as unconcerned about pet overpopulation as you are, it is very possible that by the end of one year your one cat will have progeny of twelve. At the end of two years, the number will be sixty-six. And that's only one cat. Think of it this way: if your cat doesn't have kittens, that's six less kittens we have to worry about and six less kittens that will end up abused or discarded. No, they may not be your six kittens. But believe me, because you did find homes for your kittens, there will be six kittens right here that we won't be able to find homes for.

"And that's only six kittens. The total numbers are a lot more staggering. Authorities estimate that up to ten million cats and dogs are euthanized every year in this country. Today alone, as many as 27,397 animals will die in animal shelters. Many more will die on city streets or on country roads or in research laboratories. (It's hard to reduce wasteful or repetitive animal research when scientists have an endless and cheap supply of animal subjects.) And your 'good homes' are some of our best customers. Many people thoughtlessly accept a puppy or kitten from a friend, relative, or neighbor only to turn around six months later and give the animal up at an animal shelter. (One study suggests that as many as fifty percent of the animals come in this way.) Only by the time we get him, that 'puppy' or that 'kitten' isn't cute anymore, he isn't little anymore, and he may not even be nice anymore. So you may have solved your pet overpopulation problem, but you've only compounded ours.

"Perhaps you have no intention of ever allowing your animals to breed. You keep your cat inside, and your dog is protected by a secure fence and walked on a leash. Good for you! But we still need you to sterilize your pets. Animals get loose—even those as protected as yours. Dogs have been known to jump into or out of fenced yards to get to a female in heat. And cats can be pretty ingenious and headstrong when nature calls. Even you may not be able to control your animal when it really counts. And one 'accident' is all it takes for us to be plagued with a whole new generation of unwanted animals. Wouldn't it be nice to know positively that you will never be contributing to pet overpopulation?

"And don't be a chauvinist! Male animals absolutely need to be neutered just as females need to be spayed. If you own male animals and ignore this fact, we will never be able to solve the problem of pet overpopulation.

"We can work night and day and not make a dent in pet overpopulation unless you sterilize your animal. We can't do it without you. That's why we can't stop talking about it. And we can't stop hoping that one more person will sterilize his pet so that fewer animals will be mistreated or destroyed.

"Will you be that person!"

I HAVE TRIED to find Christine Donovan for decades. I want to tell her she is a wonderful, thoughtful writer. I had thought she was with a humane society somewhere in California, years ago, when she wrote the above piece entitled: "Spaying and Neutering: Why We Can't Stop Talking about it." It could possibly have come from the Humane Society of the United States. I don't know where I got it. I just know I couldn't begin to count the thousands of copies we have printed and handed out at animal events, garage sales, rabies clinics and, on a daily basis, at the Animal Birth Control Clinic.

Only recently, I insisted on tucking a copy in a pet owner's aftercare instructions for his small dog that had just been neutered. When this man came in the front door of the clinic, he was dressed in camouflage clothing, and sported a full beard. He looked to be a real man's man. I was thinking to myself that a pit bull would surely come out of the surgery area, and this might be a person we would have to convince to keep his dog indoors for recovery from its surgery. Then, Susan, a clinic employee, brought out his small Chihuahua-poodle mix, and his reunion with his dog could not have been more dramatic. As he bundled up the still-drowsy, little dog in a soft, colorful blanket, he repeatedly kissed it on the head—and spoke to it in baby talk.

Okay. I had been wrong. It happens! Never judge a book by its cover.

The man obviously loves the heck out of his little dog—as well as the others he has at home. But then we began to talk. This loving pet owner told us about litter after litter his dogs have produced, and that the newest litter, the mama dog and puppies that were at home, was a result of a mating with the male dog he had just had neutered.

I didn't know where to begin. I climbed on my soap box, as I am so readily inclined to do. I pointed out that Lawton has a stiff mandatory neuter/spay law, and that he might very well have trouble transferring the puppies to other homes without a permit, which would be required to accompany any ad he might place in a newspaper or on a bulletin board, or anywhere else in Lawton. Finally, I assured him we were not in the habit of reporting people like himself to animal control, however, he should see to it that all the pets in his home are neutered and spayed. I think—I hope—he was convinced.

I gathered up every piece of literature and especially Christine Donovan's piece in an attempt to educate this man, who obviously cared deeply about animals, yet was, unwittingly, doing so much to contribute to their demise.

YES, MY DEAR unknown friend, Christine. We can never, ever stop talking about neutering and spaying; but we haven't even begun to start talking about pet breeding.

So, hopefully, Christine, wherever you are, just maybe you can put your wonderful writing skills to work for yet another article and entitle this one: "The Tragedy of Pet Breeding in America and Why We Must Never, Ever Stop Talking About It!"

CHAPTER 48

"You grew up, became a man, had to adjust to taking less than you hoped for; you discovered the dream machine had a big OUT OF ORDER sign on it." — Stephen King, *Dreamcatcher*

I LOVED THE Phoenix sunshine. I loved the Phoenix Suns. I loved everything about Phoenix. I thought I had landed in the promised land. I was mistaken, of course. Where pet overpopulation is concerned, there is no promised land—except perhaps in Alta, Utah.

Dan and I, and as many in our family as we could convince to go with us, moved to Phoenix in mid or late 1995. He sold the dealership in March of that same year, after twenty years. He had received a Longevity Award from Nissan as one of the longest active dealers in the United States at that time.

I didn't see stray dogs in Phoenix—except for one pit bull that would come into our lives years later. I did see a stray cactus, occasionally, which, in the distance, I would mistake for a stray dog.

There was nothing wrong with my eyes. It was just that my brain had been programmed by all those years of stray dogs and cats on roads and highways in Oklahoma—and on the road in front of my home. I seemed to be the "go-to" person for people with animal problems in my neighborhood, and in Lawton in general.

No matter where I went, someone, somewhere had to tell me their animal stories.

"I have a cute story for you," Carl said with a smile. Carl owns the gas station that services my car.

"Yeah. And what's that?" I asked politely.

Carl told me that a few days earlier he had been out to the land he leases for hunting. In an old building on the land, he had discovered a pit bull dog with puppies. One of the puppies lay dead as a huge rattlesnake was moving about them. One side of the face of the mother dog, who ran away from Carl, was tremendously swollen. The rattlesnake had played havoc with the mother and at least one of the puppies.

I was horrified. "How in the hell is this a cute story?"

Carl continued to explain to me that his daughter had rescued the two remaining puppies who were alive. He proceeded to proudly produce pictures of the puppies on his cell phone.

All I could think about was the puppies' mother. What had happened to her? Carl promised he had put food down for her, but I don't know if he went back to check on her or not. My guess would be the rattlesnake bite took her life in a slow, painful way.

My friend Carl is a good guy. A few years ago, he singlehandedly leaned on the district attorney to bring charges against a farmer for cruelty to horses. His daughter did save the lives of two adorable puppies. Carl saw the glass as half-full. I saw a dog, burdened with puppies, abandoned and frightened in a desolate pasture, trying to survive. I saw the glass as hopelessly empty.

At my granddaughter's christening, a complete stranger approached me at the church pleading for me to find a home for a dog they didn't want any longer. A complete stranger!

Is it any wonder I had to get away from this town?

How could I forget about the call I received a few years ago from a neighbor, who lives about a mile away, who wanted me to take a stray pit bull that had been "dumped out" by his house. He claimed to have kept her in a pen for four days, hoping an owner might show up.

When he brought her to the clinic, the dog had milk to indicate puppies somewhere. But where? The neighbor swore he looked for puppies and didn't see any, but if he had her penned up, would she had been able to get to them. I called him three times to quiz him on whether or not he was sure this dog had not been abandoned with puppies. He swore she hadn't.

No sooner did we get her in the clinic than Susan discovered that she had severe diarrhea in the form of pure blood. There were bones in the blood, an indication that she may have been fed chicken bones, or she had eaten road kill, We took this loving, gentle dog to a full-service veterinarian, who observed her as she passed the rest of the bones. The next day she was eating well, her diarrhea was gone, and we brought her back to the clinic.

What was this dog's story? Was she a breeding machine, and "dumped" as she was getting too old to be fully productive any longer? We will never know. These animals have no voice; they have no choice. On thing is for certain She had not had a good life. She was, most likely indoors, on a plush dog bed with a blanket, for the first time in her life, where food was good–and plentiful.

I don't remember exactly what this dog's ultimate destiny was. I don't think we found her a home. All I know is that while she lived with us, she was dearly loved and treated like royalty, compared to the life she had had.

Just this morning, as I write this book, on a Sunday, my daughter, Jamie, received a text meant for me, from a young woman, who is probably in her late thirties or early forties, whose name is Kim. I knew of Kim because she worked for a very short time in my son's law office in Oklahoma City. A year ago, my two daughters, Dana and Jamie, learned that Kim had a dog whose name was Tyson, and they were led to believe that Tyson was somewhere in Oklahoma City, and not being cared for properly.

Dana asked me if we could bring the dog to Lawton to the clinic. Once I know of an animal's plight, I can never say "no."

As it turned out, Tyson was running the streets of Harrah, Oklahoma, (wherever the hell that is), because Kim had left him there when she moved to Oklahoma City with her nineteen-year-old boyfriend's parents, who would not allow the dog in their home—or even in their back yard.

After obtaining directions to Harrah, Dana and Jamie set out to rescue Tyson. Unfortunately, he had been on his own too long and was afraid of those who were trying to help him. Kim agreed to go to Harrah and bring the dog to Lawton.

Tyson was a pit bull, boxer mix with beautiful brindle markings and a white chest. He loved people, but he had a thing for cats. He wanted to kill them. He would have loved nothing more than to gain access to our cat room where we house six to ten stray cats at any given time. For all the months that Tyson stayed with us, we had a fear he would one day find a way to get to the cats.

Tyson was also an escape artist. On multiple occasions, he would jump a six-foot wall that surrounds the back yard at the clinic. But Tyson knew where to find the hand that fed him. He knew where the arms were that hugged him. He knew the hearts who loved him, with all his mischief, were right inside that red brick building; and it didn't take him two minutes to show up at the front door waiting to get back inside his newly discovered sanctuary.

Jamie went to the clinic daily for weeks to walk Tyson and Sammy, another pit bull whose owner had also abandoned him at the clinic. (God, does it never end?)

We asked the humane society to list Tyson on their website for adoption. Kim had signed a release form giving us ownership of Tyson, however, she claimed she wanted him back. But, with her track record, we would never have given the dog back to her.

What would happen six months down the road when she failed to pay the rent and had to move. Would Tyson again be left to run the neighborhood? This is the problem with the no-kill movement and pet adoptions. It is often a revolving door of animal abandonment.

After months, when no one even came to look at Tyson or Sammie, both dogs were lovingly euthanized. The few kennels we have in what is a veterinary clinic—not a shelter—were full. We had done all we could. In the first week we had Tyson, I had personally given Kim $500 as a deposit on a rental in Oklahoma City in order for her to provide a home for her dog. That never materialized. I never wanted to see this dog put to sleep. I have never wanted to see any dog put to sleep! We have a people problem—not an animal problem—in this country.

Now, a year later, a text pops up on my cell phone. It was from Kim forwarded to me by Jamie. "This is Kim. I was wondering if u still had tyson. I have a place now and a car so I can take him thank u," said the text.

I texted back. "Tell her no, we do not have Tyson."

This was unsettling. What should I tell her? It had been a full year since we had gotten Tyson off the streets of Harrah, and months since we had had a word from his former owner.

Should I tell her a little white lie? Should I tell her we found him a good home?

What was I thinking? Hell, no! I won't lie. Why shouldn't she share the heartache we had shared by putting Tyson down? Who did she think she was to casually text us a year down the road to see if we were still accepting her responsibility for a dog she had abandoned!

My next text read: "Tell her he was euthanized and that is what happens when people get dogs they cannot take care of. We don't have room for everyone's dog. The humane society had him on their website forever but no home came up. Does she think someone else should be responsible for her dog for a year, and she just all of a sudden comes back for a dog she deserted in Harrah. We are not a shelter. We are a vet clinic. He was loved and put down kindly. We did more for the dog than she did. I gave her $500 to find a place for the dog and she did not. We all did the best we could for her dog. She failed. Not us!"

As I remembered Tyson, my anger intensified.

"Tell her the reason millions of dogs die in this country every year is because of people like her—not because of me and the clinic employees. If she really loved her dog she would have gotten him a week later like she said she was going to."

Yes, I had been blunt with Kim. Heartlessly blunt! I had given her the "unadulterated truth, stripped of any veneer," as my friend Ed Duvin had suggested in his article, "In the Name of Mercy."

This is a direct result of pet breeding. I refuse to apologize for the sins of others.

I HAD HEARD for years that Californians have a saying that "Oklahoma has the dumbest people and the most dogs." That surely is a reference to our infamous puppy mills. I, sometimes, was ashamed to say I was from Oklahoma. Once, on a flight from Oklahoma City to Phoenix, a fellow passenger asked where I was from.

"Phoenix," I said proudly.

Ok. I fudged a little, but it actually was the truth. I was from Phoenix at that moment in time, even if I didn't reveal that my roots were buried deep in Oklahoma soil.

I saw stay cats around restaurants in the tourist district of Old Town Scottsdale; but I would be told by a waiter, or a maitre d', that the cats were all spayed and neutered by the rescue groups, and most of the restaurants and businesses agreed to feed them daily. It was a cooperative effort. It was an early version of TNR, trap, neuter, release, that has become so popular today.

Lawton's animal welfare division, under the supervision of Rose Wilson, was against this form of feral cat control, and had long supported a law that makes it illegal to feed stray cats, although most people still did. The controversy that resulted when an older couple received a tremendously expensive fine for feeding cats on their own property was the catalyst, believe it or not, that brought about the Lawton 2007 mandatory neuter/spay law—and brought me back to Lawton for good.

Dan was not happy in Phoenix. He felt restrained as a businessman. He didn't know anyone there, and he knew everyone in Lawton. He liked to have coffee with other businessmen and talk shop. He was like a fish out of water—a fish in the desert. I liked it that I didn't know anyone—that no one would be calling me to take care of their animal problems. The cause of animal welfare, the arrest, and the trials had sucked the life out of me. I was exhausted and depressed. I felt helpless and hopeless.

By this time, we had neutered and spayed thousands of animals, but pet overpopulation and animal abandonment continued unabated. We were just dancing the dance. I had no strength left to try and take NOPO and the war on pet breeding national. No matter how unhappy Dan was, I, selfishly, would never agree to go back to Oklahoma. And, as ususal, he let me have my way.

We still, however, had business interests in Lawton, which brought Dan back frequently. It was what had brought him back in December, 1998.

CHAPTER 49

"When you have a sorrow that is too great, it leaves no room for any other." — Emile Zola, French writer, 1840-1902

"HI. WHAT ARE you doing?" I asked Dan over the phone.

My husband's voice—from a thousand miles away—sounded weak and tired. "I don't feel very good," he told me. "I've been in bed most of the afternoon."

It was December 10, 1998. He was at the house in Oklahoma. I was in Phoenix.

We landed in Phoenix because Dan had a sister who lived there, and she had convinced us to purchase a small condominium in Scottsdale just a few blocks from her house. We had visited there occasionally while still living in Oklahoma. We sold the condo and purchased a larger house a few months later, this time in Paradise Valley, another Phoenix suburb. I would move at least three more times, before settling in a home in Ahwatukee, a suburb in the East Valley, just two doors away from my two grandchildren.

We still had business interests in Oklahoma, which brought Dan back frequently. We couldn't bear to sell our home, even though now it was a shell of a home. We had taken most of the furniture to Phoenix, leaving only a couple of beds, the kitchen table and other bits here and there. The house rang of emptiness.

"I feel sorry for the house," Dan would say as we would pull out of the drive to return to Phoenix. I rarely would come back to Lawton with Dan on those business trips. We had a large RV which made it easy to transport all the animals back and forth, but I didn't want to come back.

On those occasions when I did come with him, we would walk into the big, lonely house that sat almost at the edge of a creek bank, and open a bottle of wine at the battered old chopping block that sat in the middle of the kitchen floor. We both would declare our love for this old house, and the dogs were thrilled to be "home." And I would wonder, momentarily, why we were now calling the strange land in the desert home.

After we had been in Lawton, however, for two or three days, I would have a change of heart. "Have I told you how much I hate this town?" I would ask, as

Dan and I would be driving down a Lawton street. He would laugh at me. I had said it so many times.

Two of my five grandchildren were in Phoenix, but three grandsons were in Oklahoma City. I had pangs of guilt about not spending more time with the three in Oklahoma. I have that guilt to this day.

In fact, burdening myself with guilt is an old familiar trait of mine. I was not only guilty of leaving three of my grandchildren in Oklahoma while I lived in Phoenix. I was guilty of leaving the Animal Birth Control Clinic and the humane society for Linda to oversee—almost singlehandedly.

I had, sadly enough, been brought back to Oklahoma in 1996 by the death of my nephew who suffered from severe bi-polar disease and had taken his own life. His father—my brother—was diagnosed with lung cancer, and seemed to have no will to fight it, and was dead in 1997, within seven months of burying his son. My 92-year-old mother had died in January of 1995, two months before Dan sold the dealership. We would never have moved to Phoenix if she had still been alive. I had lost three family members in three years.

I have never forgotten the strange statement my sister from California had made while we were sitting in the funeral car at my brother's funeral.

"I wonder who'll be next," she had said.

IN THIRTY MINUTES, I made another call to Dan.

"How are you feeling now?" I asked.

"I'm in the kitchen looking for an aspirin. Don't think we have any, but I found a bottle of Tylenol. I'm gonna take a couple and go back to bed," he said.

"I was going to try to come back to Phoenix today, "Dan told me, "but I couldn't find anyone to take me to the airport."

Even though Lawton has an airport, we always went to Oklahoma City, about an hour away, for direct flights to Phoenix.

"I'll be coming home tomorrow, for sure," Dan said. "This guy I know is going to take me to the airport. I don't know why I can't think of his name. I wrote his phone number down on a piece of paper."

The longer I talked to Dan, the more concerned I became. Something was just not right.

"Tell me the phone number," I said.

Dan read the phone number on the piece of paper to me. I recognized the number immediately. It was Linda and Dayman's phone number.

These were people who were neighbors and friends for thirty years. We had partied with them, rescued trailers full of dogs with them, played cards with them, had barbeques with them. Linda and I had been together through hell and back in the cause of animal welfare.

And now my husband couldn't remember Dayman's name! This was frightening. I knew something was terribly wrong.

"Dan," I said, "that's Dayman's number. You could be having a stroke. You need to go to the hospital."

He was adamant that he wouldn't go to the hospital.

"Then just let me call Mildred to come out and stay with you for a while," I pleaded.

Mildred had worked for us as a housekeeper and was caretaker of our pets when we were away. She was also a dear friend and we thought of her as family.

"No," Dan said firmly. "Don't call Mildred. I don't want anyone out here," he insisted. "I'm just going to take these Tylenols and go to bed."

Reluctantly, I agreed. "OK," I said. "But I will be calling you again in 30 minutes, or sooner, to check on you, so don't get mad at me for calling so often. I'm worried about you."

I don't think I waited another thirty minutes. Probably twenty minutes later, I called the house again. The house phone was on the night stand right beside the bed. It rang once, twice, three times—and over and over again. There was no answer.

I was panicked. I called our closest neighbor across the street and asked if he would go look at the driveway to see if Dan's car was in the drive.

He reported back to me that the car was there.

My next call was to Mildred. She had a key to the house, and a remote to the front gate. She was the obvious person to be able to get inside the house. She assured me she would go, but she was going to ask a male friend to go with her as, I think, she was afraid of what she was going to find.

I called my son, Monty, in Oklahoma City. Our other three children were in Phoenix. Monty, most likely, endangered his own life driving at breakneck speed, enough so to attract the attention of an Oklahoma Highway Patrol unit, which proved to be a blessing in that the officer escorted him to Lawton.

I called Dayman who agreed to go to the house, and look inside the large sliding glass door of the bedroom. He was able to see Dan lying on the bed, but unable to awaken him by pounding on the glass and calling out to him.

Someone called an ambulance. I'm not sure who it was. By now, Mildred and her friend had unlocked the house and were waiting for the ambulance to arrive.

Monty made it to the hospital at about the same time the ambulance was arriving. He called me in Phoenix.

"It doesn't look good, mom," he told me.

I had already started calling airlines. By now it was around nine o'clock in the evening. The last Southwest flight left Phoenix around 6:00 p.m. I even called a couple of people in Phoenix who I knew might possibly know someone who had a private plane. The best available flight was on American at 2:00 a.m. to Dallas. That was as close as we could get to Lawton. My youngest son, Paul, who also lived in Phoenix, booked the flight for me, for himself, and for my two daughters. His wife stayed in Phoenix to care for their two children and everyone's dogs and cats.

I was in a daze. I found one of Dan's old flannel work shirts, that hadn't been laundered—making it even more special—and I wore it on the flight, and for days in the hospital.

Dan had suffered a brain hemorrhage on the right side of his brain. He was unable to talk, but Monty and the doctors believed that, for a couple of hours, right after the incident, he was able to hear what was being said to him. Monty was telling him how much we all loved him, and that "mom is on the way."

Monty told me that a tear had rolled down his cheek which was an indication he had heard. The flight from Phoenix to Dallas was about two hours. Paul's lifelong friend, Tom Ballesteri, who lives in Ft.Worth, picked us up at DFW, and drove us to Lawton—another two to three hours. That was the longest trip from Phoenix to Lawton that I could ever remember—even longer than those fourteen-hour road trips with all the animals.

By the time I got to the ICU unit at the hospital, Dan was brain dead. We wouldn't accept that he couldn't hear us. Daily, we pleaded into his ear, asking him to "please wake up." Monty brought in a CD player with music by Pavoratti, Bocelli, and other Italian greats, and placed it next to his ear in hopes of a response.

Finally, in an attempt to make us realize that Dan was gone, the doctors ordered a test. They would take him off life support to show us there was no brain activity. The test was done. The doctors were right. Dan was brain dead.

On December 16, we agreed that the life support would be removed. The love of my life, and the biggest supporter in anything I had ever attempted, was gone.

Oddly enough, Dan's sister had died a few years earlier at the exact same age—age sixty-two—of the exact same malady. It was a genetic condition, one that we knew nothing about.

While Dan had been hospitalized those six days, streams of well-wishers had flooded into the hallway of that hospital. But even on the occasion of my husband's death, however, I was unable to escape an animal incident. The event seems almost like an out-of-body experience and I have, for years, asked myself if it is even true—or, if somehow, I merely imagined it.

Obviously, there had been an automobile accident or a police stop of an automobile that had a dog on board. I was approached in the intensive care unit of the hospital by an officer who inquired as to what they should do with the puppy. I don't know for sure how I responded, but I was in no position to help with their animal problem at that time.

I had no idea Dan had touched so many people's lives. All his former employees had come to the hospital. Dan Mullins, who had purchased the Nissan dealership, didn't miss a day at the hospital, and scores of people, some of whom I didn't even know, came to see if there was something they could do. The local chapter of the NAACP, of which Dan and I had become lifetime members, honored Dan with a resolution at his funeral. Even the local television station acknowledged his life and death.

And here I was, back in Lawton—that town I had come to hate—and I had never seen a larger outpouring of love from a community as was shown to my husband at the time of his death.

In fact, a strange thing happened as the funeral procession headed for the cemetery, escorted by the Lawton Police Department. I was riding in the funeral car, and as the funeral procession rounded the corner at an intersection, a police officer stood at attention and saluted the hearse that carried my husband to the cemetery.

Days later, I asked the director of the funeral home if that salute by the Lawton policeman was standard procedure.

"I have never seen that before in my life," he told me. That was significant! Truly significant!

TWO DAYS BEFORE CHRISTMAS, I found myself wandering the aisles of Walmart, one of my least favorite places to be in the world. I mindlessly filled a shopping cart with groceries.

Tom had brought out a fresh Christmas tree, and the earthy smell of fresh pine filled the half-empty living room.

Five grandchildren, ranging from three to eight years old, were waiting for Christmas.

WHEN I WAS able to gather my thoughts and somehow find adequate words to express my appreciation, I purchased an ad in the Lawton Constitution acknowledging all the kindness shown to our family at the most difficult time of our lives.

"Dan Delluomo brought so much into the lives of his family and friends," I wrote. "He was a kind and patient man, who will be remembered for his jovial, down-to-earth manner, his cheerful smile and, to those of us who knew him best, for his gentle nature and quiet generosity that extended not only to humans but to animals as well."

I thanked friends, doctors and nurses, pall bearers, the NAACP, the staff at Channel 7, the ministers, the funeral home director, and everyone I could remember who had been so kind to us. And, finally, I thanked the Lawton Police Department for "escorting Dan to his final resting place, with a special word of gratitude to the officer, who stood at attention and saluted, as the hearse drove by. We saw your gesture and we thank you. Dan surely saw you, too. He must have smiled.

"And now as we face our tomorrows without our beloved Dan, but forever with his spirit and our precious memories, we are comforted in the knowledge of God's continued love for us and, because of your kindness, by a renewed sense of the meaning of family and friendship.

"Thank you again for what you've meant to Dan and what you continue to mean to us. We are eternally grateful."

I had made my peace with my hometown. But like a ship in uncharted waters, I was lost. I didn't know where I belonged. I wouldn't know for years.

CHAPTER 50

"I've missed more than 9000 shots in my career. I've lost almost 300 games. Twenty-six times, I've been trusted to take the game winning shot and missed. I've failed over and over and over again in my life. And that is why I succeed." — Michael Jordan

I DIDN'T COMPLETELY abandon the animal cause when we moved to Phoenix. Because I wasn't continually chasing stray dogs and cats, I had more time for using my brain rather than my brawn.

I got myself together enough to get the NOPO video aired on public access TV, and on one occasion when I was in downtown Phoenix, on a whim, I visited the office of the infamous Sheriff Joe Arpaio.

Before I knew anything about the sheriff's controversial politics, I had seen him on television declaring how animal cruelty of any kind would not be tolerated in Maricopa County. To say I was impressed was an understatement. I had come from a state where the vast majority of county law enforcement officials weren't even aware that animal cruelty laws existed—let alone enforce them.

Arpaio had created the Animal Crimes Investigations Unit, apparently one of the few of its kind in the nation, and seized animals were cared for in the Maricopa County Sheriff's Safe Haven (MASH) unit, which included a grooming parlor staffed by inmates.

The sheriff actually met with me, and I shared with him my thoughts about pet overpopulation and breeding laws. He was polite, receptive, and even suggested to his secretary that I had "good ideas."

Yes, I was like a Mormon without a bicycle—preaching the neuter/spay and anti-breeding brand of religion wherever I could find an ear to listen.

It was also during those first couple of years we were in Phoenix that I wrote all those letters to celebrities. I mentioned earlier about my bizarre letter to Hustler Magazine publisher Larry Flint.

"So, it would seem to me," I wrote at the end of my letter to Mr. Flint, "if the man who has promoted sex in humans began a crusade to stop sex in dogs and cats . . . what a stir it would create—and that is exactly what we need. A big huge national stir! I told Mr. Flint we need people to understand how vital it is that they adopt from animal shelters rather than buying from pet shops and breeders.

I never heard from Larry Flint.

I wrote to Maury Povich. His show seemed to thrive on controversy. I received a postcard advising me that my "Segment Idea" would be reviewed at an upcoming producer's meeting.

"I am encouraged that this idea will be reviewed at your producer's meeting and take that as a glimmer of hope that it will seriously be considered for a show. I am certain, beyond a shadow of a doubt, that if it is controversy you are looking for, place breeders on one side of the issue, and animal shelter workers who have killed too many pets, or those who have busted puppy mills, on the other, and I assure you tempers will flare. And rightfully so. As I said to you in a previous letter, pet breeders are pimps . . ."

I wrote that "people become very emotional about animals and animal cruelty, and I believe a show on this topic would knock the competition out of the water."

Obviously, the producers of the show didn't agree with me. I never heard from them. On May 6, 1997, I sent a fax referencing "A war on pet breeding and puppy mills in the U.S." to *The Montel Williams Show*. It read: "If you want pathetic video footage of puppy mills in Kansas and Oklahoma, please call Deloris. I can make tape after tape available to you. You will then have no doubt as to why a war should be waged on pet breeding."

In my letter to Mr. Williams, I told him if he wanted "controversy on your show, believe me, this is it. Just get a group of breeders or American Kennel Club VPs on one side and some shelter workers . . . on the other, and watch the fur fly (no pun intended)!"

I never heard from *The Montel Williams Show*.

I wrote to Ms. Wendy Morris of PMK Public Relations, who represented Mary Tyler Moore. I was requesting Ms. Moore consider being a spokesperson for NOPO.

I explained that our campaign required a spokesperson who would not be intimidated by the controversy that would "undoubtedly be created by greedy breeders and the American Kennel Club, who fight tooth and nail against any campaigns to slow pet breeding. They line their pockets as animals die physically, and those who kill them die emotionally, as has happened to many of us involved in this cause.

"The issue is so tragic and in-depth, it is impossible to explain in this space," I wrote. I told Ms. Morris we have rolls and rolls of puppy mill footage taken by TV stations in Kansas and Oklahoma.

I also wrote a letter to Mary Tyler Moore herself.

"On June 2, 1997, I sent you three videos depicting the horrors of puppy mills in Oklahoma, as well as a video on euthanasia of pets in animal shelters.

" . . . We need a celebrity of your magnitude to free these innocent pets from their kennels from hell. "Imagine the hell these animals live in for their entire lives . . . all because uninformed Americans continue to buy pets from pet shops where these puppies wind up (if they live long enough)."

I made a fool of myself. I begged. "Someone has to care about these forgotten animals. Please, Ms. Moore, please help . . . Please. I beg you, I implore you for their sakes. They are all but ignored by the animal rights movement. It has been going on for years."

My pleas obviously fell on deaf ears. I heard nothing from Ms. Morris or Mary Tyler Moore.

I contacted The *Sally Jesse Raphael Show, The Ricki Lake Show, The Jenny Jones Show, The Geraldo Show, The Jerry Springer Show*—all popular talk shows in the nineties. I wrote a long letter to Michael Moore.

I heard nothing. Nada. Zilch.

Michael Jordan said he has failed over and over and over again in his life; and that is why he succeeds.

If repeated failure is a guarantee of success, then we should be on the brink of something big in the battle against pet overpopulation in America!

CHAPTER 51

"Animals, like us, are living souls. They are not things. They are not objects. Neither are they human. Yet they mourn. They love. They dance. They suffer. They know the peaks and chasms of being." — Gary Kowalski, *The Souls of Animals*

"THE PIT BULL was gone this morning. The pasture and rickety old metal shed that had been her home for a month, seemed empty and still. I set out her food, as usual. This morning, her treat had been two slices of cheese on top of the canned food mixed with dry.

"Anything could have happened. She hung out too often in the middle of the road. She could have been hit. But where was her body? I have searched the ditches on both sides of the road.

"Could she have been shot by a farmer? I seriously don't know. I had been given permission by a neighbor to feed the dog on his property, and to place bedding and hay in the old metal shed where she took refuge. Her body print was still in the thick, round dog bed I had placed in the middle of the pile of soft hay.

"There is a remote, very remote, possibility that someone stopped for her and was able to pick her up, but I had been unable to gain her trust enough to come to me, so I doubt she would have trusted anyone else.

"I was able to get within a few feet from her, but human beings had failed her, and she trusted no one—not even the hand that fed her.

"I saw a coyote at her food bowl yesterday morning. Could she have taken up with the coyotes? That has been my fear. She could probably have held her own with one of them, but did they gang up on her and kill her?

"Perhaps she is in heat and running the county. I don't know. I don't know where she is. I just know that she's gone.

"Today is my birthday, and I am tired of nothing changing as I age."

I HAVE NEVER maintained a diary or a journal in my entire life. For some reason I can't explain, when I came home from taking fresh food about a mile up the road to a pit bull I had been feeding twice a day, for at least a month, something compelled me to sit down and write the above words.

Linda had helped me set out a large trap to try and catch the white pit bull with brown markings. But the damn trap was old and it malfunctioned. When the trap snapped shut—without her in it—I'm sure it frightened her, and I was afraid she might never come back. But she did. She came back every day for the next two weeks. I continued to take her food twice a day. We had a routine. I would pull up to the pasture gate, call out to her, and honk my horn. I could see her standing in a rusted-out opening in the small, dilapidated tin shed, peering out at me.

I think she desperately wanted to trust me. As soon as I would drive away, she would amble slowly, cautiously, down to the gate and eat her food.

But now, like so many other abandoned and helpless animals, she was gone, without a trace, in spite of my best efforts to help her.

There had been so many other stray pit bulls. But, somehow, this one was special.

Perhaps she reminded me of Pumpkin.

I FOUND SOLACE in my anonymity in the fifth largest city in the nation. I foolishly believed I was living in a Utopian community, where people were better educated, more financially sound, and, therefore, dogs and cats were better cared for and not often abandoned.

I knew, however, deep in my soul, there were neighborhoods in which I should never travel and, on one occasion when I did, I learned the hard way that Phoenix is no different than Lawton or any other city, large or small, when it comes to pet overpopulation in America. Because of that trip to that neighborhood, our lives would be in turmoil; and I would lose the anonymity that I cherished in Ahwatukee, my quiet little suburb of Phoenix—at least, for a period of time.

AFTER DAN'S DEATH, I was a lost soul. I was forced to make regular trips back to Lawton for those same business reasons that had brought him back. Now I had to make a living.

When I was in Phoenix, a simple country landscape scene in a movie would make me long for my home in Oklahoma. When I came home without Dan, however, the unbearable loneliness would consume me, and I would load up the animals and head back, once again, to Phoenix. I didn't know where I belonged, or where I wanted to belong.

I just happened to be in Oklahoma on April 18, 2008, when I received a phone call from Jamie in Phoenix. She was crying uncontrollably into the phone. "Mom, I am in so much trouble."

Maricopa County Animal Care and Control officers were at her home, and in the process of taking her three dogs, Lucy, a Boston terrier/pit bull mix, Boomer, a bassett hound mix, and Pumpkin, an American Staffordshire terrier aka a pit bull, to the Maricopa County Animal Shelter.

Jamie was hysterical. It was hard for me to piece together what she was trying to tell me. Although she had not let me know, the previous day a terrible accident had happened involving her dogs while she was out on a walk. Jamie has been walking her dogs for years from three to five miles a day. It's almost an obsession with her to this day.

Phoenix is a dog-walking community, and Jamie was always careful when walking the dogs. She had to contain their excitement, by tightening up on their leashes, when they saw a rabbit. She made sure, as a precautionary measure, to turn around and walk in a different direction when she observed another person with dogs.

On that particular morning in April, Jamie was not feeling well and had stopped to rest in one of the area green belts. She and the three dogs were relaxing in the shade of a mesquite tree, and she had answered a quick cell phone call. She had the dogs' leashes secured in her hand when, all of a sudden, a woman with two small Yorkies approached the area. Jamie had often seen this woman on her walks and had always avoided her. The woman knew there was a pit bull, and a Boston terrier/pit bull mix, close by the area she was approaching. I will never understand why she would have chosen that path. She had deliberately crossed the street from where she was walking to pursue a path that would take her and her tiny Yorkies directly in front of a huge pit bull and two other dogs.

When the small Yorkies approached the area where Jamie and her dogs were resting, Jamie's dogs lunged forward, breaking loose from the leashes that were clipped together. The three dogs, led by Pumpkin, went after the Yorkies. Jamie was in pursuit of her dogs, but before she could reach them, Pumpkin had already attacked the Yorkies. And Lucy and Boomer were involving themselves in the mix.

Christine Meyers, the Yorkies' owner, reached down to protect her dogs, and in the process her arm was bitten. Jamie also tried to grab the Yorkies and was bitten by one of them, and, at the same time, had fallen in a huge cactus resulting in thorns all over her ankles. It was a bloody scene, to say the least.

Ms. Meyers went to the hospital to have her arm treated and Nora, the Yorkie who had suffered the worst injuries, went to the veterinarian, but was returned home the same day. Both dogs survived and, to the best of my knowledge, have not suffered any long term effects from the tragic event.

Animal control impounded all three of Jamie's dogs, claiming they couldn't be sure which one had bit Ms. Meyers.

"Dog in mauling to be destroyed," was the headline and the lead front page story of the Ahwatukee Foothills News on May 7.

"Phoenix Municipal Court Judge Gloria Ybarra has ordered Pumpkin be destroyed," wrote Doug Murphy, staff writer for the paper.

"By all accounts, people who know the pit bull, and the two others that Jamie Delluomo was walking near Kyrene de la Esperanza Elementary School April 17, are usually calm, stable dogs." Murphy quoted a dog trainer that we had asked to evaluate the dogs as being "very nice, sweet, affectionate dogs."

Murphy's articles about Pumpkin, however, were laced with mistakes, and, in my opinion, were biased. He erroneously referred to Pumpkin as "he" and wrote that all of Jamie's dogs were pit bulls. It was interesting that a reporter, who should have been objective in a matter on which he was reporting, sat next to Ms. Meyers in the courtroom.

After Pumpkin was euthanaized, Murphy wrote that I defended Pumpkin to the end, and that I was "bitter at the legal process, despite having an attorney and a two-day hearing in Phoenix Municipal Court."

Murphy wrote that I "complained that (Judge) Ybarra rushed the second day of testimony because she was going on vacation for two weeks . . ."

That was true. The hearing was set for 2:00 p.m. on May 1, but started late and ended at 5:00 p.m. to reconvene at 9:00 a.m. the following day, but started late again. At around 11:00 a.m. Judge Ybarra announced she had to leave at 11:30 to go to her daughter's graduation and wouldn't return until May 13. That amounted to approximately three hours of court time.

Jamie, by this time, had cashed in her 401K and was broke. She had paid for little Nora's veterinarian bill, and was forced to hire a lawyer; she was paying $100 per day in shelter fees; and the judge had to leave for thirteen days before she could make a decision as to whether or not Pumpkin should be destroyed?

The judge, however, made a decision that afternoon outside the courtroom and relayed it by phone or fax, and there was no chance to plead for a different outcome for Pumpkin.

On the day of Pumpkin's death, Jamie received notice she was being sued by Ms. Meyers and it was interesting that the Ahwatukee Foothills News, who had reported Pumpkin's incident and euthanasia so widely, made no mention of the lawsuit. I also found it interesting that the lawyer for Ms. Meyers was a regular advertiser in the publication.

This "pit bull" incident created a huge controversy as pit bull stories always do. Animal rights activists all over Phoenix weighed in on the subject, especially after the Ahwatukee newspaper published an unbelievable editorial entitled: "Pit bulls unfit as family pets," by staff writer Emily Behrendt.

"Ahwatukee Foothills is such a passionately dog-loving community, it's always sad to hear when a furry companion attacks one of our own," wrote Behrendt.

"And, admit it, it came as no surprise that the canine assailant turned out to be a pit bull. "Earlier this week, a ruling by Phoenix Municipal Court ordered Pumpkin the pit bull to be euthanized for attacking and seriously injuring Ahwatukee Foothills resident Christene Meyers and her Yorkie, Nora, on April 17.

Why could this paper not get it right? Pumpkin did not attack Christene Meyers. I don't believe she would ever have attacked a human being outright. Ms. Meyers was injured while trying to save her Yorkie, and who could fault her for that? But Pumpkin did not attack Ms. Meyers.

"Defenders of the pit bull stigma claim that no breed is inherently dangerous, and that we should regard a dog as dangerous only if it has behaved in a dangerous manner," wrote Behrendt.

"But let's face it, certain breeds behave in a dangerous manner a lot more often than others. "Of the 32 fatal dog attacks in the United States during 2007, literally half of the named breeds were pit bulls. Nine of the victims were children ages 2 to 11. Five of the victims were elderly, ages fifty-nine and older, including ninety-year-old Celestino Rangel from San Antonio, Texas, who was killed by two pit bulls that had broken into his home and attacked him.

"These are not examples of these dogs being 'singled out,' but the hard truth that they are dangerous animals. No other breed attacks adults nearly as often as they attack children, which pit bulls do. The breed also attacks without warning and often without provocation.

"Combine the number of attacks with their enormous jaw strength, which the dogs developed over years of selective breeding, and their 'lock and shake' trait, which causes severe bone and muscle injury, pit bull owners have a very real ticking time bomb in their homes."

"Why take that chance?" Behrendt asked. "Why do people choose to put themselves, their children and their community members at risk?

"It's not just pit bulls, either; I'm talking about all violence-prone dogs.

"A study by the Animal People News tracked the number of dog attack deaths and maimings from September 1982 to November 2007. The number of pit bull incidents that inflicted bodily harm was 1,194, resulting in 116 deaths. Rottweilers came in second with 427 inflictions of bodily harm and 63 deaths, and wolf-dog hybrids came in a distant third with 79 instances of bodily harm and 19 deaths. German shepherds, chows and Akitas also topped the list.

"A lot of these instances were, no doubt, a result of improper training. The average Joe Public is not equipped with the time, knowledge or tools necessary to keep violence-prone dogs under control. But not to do so is still irresponsible.

"That's why I believe such dogs should not be adopted as family pets at all, but rather placed in homes that would better play to their strengths: Security.

"Restrict pit bull and rottweiler ownership to warehouses, factories, junk yards and other places that require safeguarding.

"Make sure they're trained by professionals who know what they are doing. Keep them properly restrained by chains that don't break.

"Keep children and seniors inaccessible to them," warned Ms. Behrendt. "And little Yorkies named Nora."

I could accept some of what was in Ms. Behrendt's opinion piece, but I had a problem with the part about junk yards, and warehouses, and keeping dogs on chains. I do know that chaining a dog only makes them more aggressive, and that is why so many communities, in this day and age, have no-chain laws. I have seen, in Oklahoma, more than one pit bill on huge tractor chains with bricks tied to them—obviously to train them to be stronger fighters.

I also know that keeping any dog at the end of a chain is one of the most inhumane practices that can be heaped on a voiceless creature!

As would be expected, pit bull, rottweiler and German shepherd owners were outraged and expressed it in their own letters to the editor.

Others wrote to agree with Ms. Behrendt.

Animal Care and Control Sgt. Gerado Elizalde was right in his statement to the newspaper. "Owners are responsible for the actions of their animals, regardless. But there are no winners in a case like this, and the loser is Pumpkin.

DR. RODRIGO SILVA, director of Maricopa County Animal Care and Control dug in on his decision to have Pumpkin destroyed, in spite of our pleas to save her. He had the power to suggest a stay of execution, but he chose against it.

Jamie had begged to be allowed to bring Pumpkin back to Oklahoma to live in the country with a six-foot wall around a five-acre yard. She offered to have Pumpkin defanged, to never walk her again, or do whatever was demanded to save her life. Animal control and the county sheriff's office in Lawton had e-mailed Silva expressing their willingness to accept her into their jurisdictions.

In spite of our efforts, and those of the animal rights community in Phoenix, to save Pumpkin, she was euthanized on May 8, 2008.

Silva's stance on the matter seemed odd. He was obviously a pit bull lover. Only two weeks after the incident and two weeks before Pumpkin was euthanized, a heartfelt, gut-wrenching letter to the editor, written by Silva, appeared in the April 30 edition of the Ahwatukee paper.

The subject matter was his love for the pit bull breed. I have always wondered if Pumpkin's case was what inspired his writing.

"As a young adult, I had an American Staffordshire Terrier, who was given up by her previous owners because she was 'too hyper,' Silva wrote.

"Tatanka, as I named her, gave me many happy, love-filled years. We were meant for each other; we hiked, jogged and played together. She was not only a companion, but also my best friend and confidant. Tatanka never hurt anyone or anything. She was a big dog with a puppy's attitude and a tear-jerking love for little kids. All the children in the neighborhood knew her by name and would play her favorite games, such as "throw the ball and never get it back," "chase me—you'll never catch me," "pin you down and lick your face," and many others.

"When Tatanka's life was senselessly taken by a poisoned piece of meat, she took with her forever a piece of my heart. I can't understand what would have made someone take the life of such a precious, loving creature. Perhaps it was fear caused by the size and stature of that awe- inspiring animal, which made that unkind heart kill that big, gentle spirit.

"Phantom heartaches stab my chest when I see the Pitbulls in our shelter. I know that most of them won't make it to the next day.

"What have we done to these beautiful dogs? Pitbulls were once the 'Nanny dog of America.' There was a time when Petey the Pitbull accompanied the Little Rascals in all their adventures, warming children's hearts throughout the nation.

"Today, many Bullies love and are loved by their families. Unfortunately, many more will lose their lives at the gentle hands of a shelter worker, who couldn't possibly find good homes for them all.

"Do you know that almost a third of all the dogs coming through the animal shelter system in the Valley are Pitbulls? Yes, you read it right; approximately 20,000 Pitbulls will find themselves in a shelter every year. Most of them are good dogs in need of a loving home.

"Pitbulls are intelligent, precocious and athletic dogs that will do nearly anything asked of them. They are hard-wired to be animal aggressive and people must be mindful of this heritage, especially around children and small animals.

"Although wonderful companions, Pitbulls are not for beginners; these are dogs that need an experienced and well-informed owner who is ready to make a commitment. They need a kind, but firm, caretaker that can funnel their gleeful zest for life through exercise, training and service. These dogs will return your care and attention ten-fold; they will always be loving and devoted to their families.

"Most of the ones we see in our shelters are there because their owners did not know what they were getting into when they acquired a Bully. Sadly, there are not enough good homes for them. These beautiful animals have a greater risk of being euthanized than any other breed. In fact, a 50 percent higher risk.

"Rescue groups don't want them as they are harder to place than any other dog. Many people don't understand the breed and are unreasonably afraid of them. Of all the Bullies in the shelter, less than 1 percent will go to a rescue group, 12 percent will be claimed by their owners, and 10 percent will be adopted. More than 73 percent will be euthanized.

"Together we need to stop the irrational breeding of Pitbulls. What can you do to save these beautiful animals? If you own a Pitbull, sterilize him, train him and socialize him. Encourage friends and family to sterilize their dogs. If you are looking for a pet, do not buy from a store, the newspaper or the backyard breeder. Adopt your new dog from the animal shelter. Volunteer to support your favorite animal shelter.

"The shelters alone cannot solve the problem. It is up to us as a community to end this tragedy."

In spite of Silva's expressed love for the pit bull breed, there was no saving Pumpkin. Did Silva see Pumpkin in that small cage in his shelter? Did the "size and stature" of this "awe-inspiring animal" remind him of his Tatanka? Did he realize that Pumpkin dearly loved people but was "hard-wired to be animal aggressive?"

Did he know that Jamie never missed a day, driving for miles to the shelter in the West Valley, where she sat on the concrete floor outside Pumpkin's cage for hours? He surely knew that Pumpkin's death would take with Jamie forever a piece of her heart, just as Tatanka's death had taken a piece of his.

Yes, Tatanka sounded a lot like Pumpkin. And Silva sounded a lot like me.

Silva did what he thought he had to do. I hold no grudges with his decision. God only knows, I, myself, have played a part in the deaths of too many pit bulls to judge him.

The one concession we were allowed was that Pumpkin could die in the compassionate environment of her veterinarian. Animal control delivered her to the clinic, where we met her, and they waited in the parking lot to be sure she was dead. Pumpkin died surrounded by people who loved her—wagging her back end in happiness at being reunited with her family. We brought her body back to Oklahoma and buried her on the banks of the creek surrounding our home.

That same day, I went to the Ahwatukee Foothill News and purchased a full page ad entitled "In Memory of Pumpkin." It was time for me to have my say.

Following are excerpts from the ad: "Pumpkin died today," I wrote. Not from any disease that plagues the canine species. Not because the family who loved her didn't fight for her. Not because countless numbers of animal welfare people we didn't even know didn't plead for her life.

"Pumpkin died today partly because we could not bear to see her continue in confinement, where she was going cage crazy, while we appealed her death sentence. Our request for her to be walked at least a short distance each day was denied. Our veterinarian's request to board her during the appeal process was denied. Our willingness to post bond if she could be moved from her small cage was denied.

" . . . So Pumpkin died. But there is a broader issue surrounding her death, and the unfortunate accident in which she was involved, than meets the eye.

"Pumpkin was a victim. She was born because an irresponsible pet owner failed to have her mother spayed and, through no fault of her own, she was a breed maligned by much of society.

"But she, nevertheless, was born. And, there she stood. A six-month old puppy, on the side of a quiet road in the industrial section of Mesa where my daughter Jamie had accompanied me to purchase cabinets for my home in Ahwatukee.

"Pumpkin, who was far too thin and had developed mange, waddled up to Jamie wagging the entire back end of her body in a way that became her most distinguishable characteristic . . . that along with the persistent licking on people around her. Pumpkin literally loved people.

"Pumpkin went home with Jamie, who took her the next day to the Arizona Humane Society because she already had Boomer, a beagle-basset mix and Lucy, a Boston terrier mix, and she didn't need another dog.

"But Jamie had fallen in love. She went back to the Humane Society and left with her new best friend in tow, along with her adoption papers which noted 'nice dog.'

"And 'nice dog' was the opinion of many who knew Pumpkin. Jamie's friends, her family, her veterinarian and staff, a professional dog trainer, and more than a few kennel workers in both Mesa and the 27th Avenue facility knew Pumpkin and the other two dogs as 'nice dogs.'

"We will always be grateful that Pumpkin was able to enjoy a wonderful life for her three short years, which is far more than millions of dogs in this country are afforded. Our daily visits to Pumpkin brought home once again an indisputable fact: We have a terrible pet overpopulation problem in this country.

"The sad eyes and the dejected demeanor of the abandoned animals we saw was nothing short of heartbreaking. We learned shelter code: OWB stands for 'owner wants back.' DNWB means 'does not want back.'

"YES," I wrote in capital letters. "THERE SHOULD BE A BAN ON THE BREEDING OF PIT BULLS! There, I said it. But before there is a rush to believe I have conceded that Pumpkin should have died, read on.

"There should also be a ban on the breeding of Yorkies, and cockers, and black labs, and Jack Russell Terriers, and Irish Setters and . . . well, you get the picture.

"These are just some of the breeds I have seen wind up in animal shelters who never found homes and were eventually euthanized.

"It is no more of a moral sin to rescue a pit bull puppy from the streets of Mesa and love it dearly than to perpetuate pet breeding by buying pets from breeders or pet shops, where most of the puppies come from the little shops of horror we call puppy mills.

"What I have learned in all these years of fighting for animals is this: We can build bigger and better shelters, where larger numbers of pets can be housed and killed, we can educate children in schools, we can neuter and spay until we're blue in the face, and try to convince those who already have too many pets to adopt just one more.

"But as long as pet owners fail to act responsibly by having their pets neutered and spayed, as long as consumers continue to encourage breeding by buying rather than adopting or rescuing, and as long as legislators fail to regulate responsibly by enacting breeding laws, no one wins.

"And beyond any doubt, the greatest losers of all are the Pumpkins and the DNWBs who pop up on roadsides and wind up in shelters for a sin no greater than simply being born.

"Today, my resolve to fight for these abandoned and helpless animals is stronger than ever and I will continue to do so—in memory of Pumpkin."

The lawsuit against Jamie was dropped inasmuch as she was living in a home that was in my name and the homeowner's policy would not cover any damages for Ms. Meyers, and Jamie was at the end of her financial resources.

The court, however, ordered Jamie to pay restitution to Ms. Meyers for medical bills. She paid that restitution for years. I, personally, spent several thousand dollars on legal fees.

This experience was just another sad example of the consequences of pet overpopulation in America.

So much for life in the promised land!

CHAPTER 52

"If one person is unkind to an animal it is considered to be cruelty, but where a lot of people are unkind to animals, especially in the name of commerce, the cruelty is condoned and, once large sums of money are at stake, will be defended to the last by otherwise intelligent people."
— Ruth Harrison, *Animal Machines*

BY 2003, I was spending most of my time back in Oklahoma. While I was in Phoenix, Linda had turned the humane society over to the new group, which is a no-kill organization and adoptions are their primary focus. They are, however, to their credit, serious neuter/spay advocates. The animal cruelty work we tried to do in the city and the county, where no animal control exists, fell by the wayside.

Without the work of the humane society, we could find more time to pursue "litter laws" which were our passion, right alongside neutering and spaying.

I can't recall what exactly prompted us to attempt the impossible: A statewide law that very much resembled a mandatory neuter/spay law. In Oklahoma? Were we delusional? In Oklahoma?

We rolled out our statewide campaign by fashioning hot pink card stock into seven-by-ten-inch postcards which carried thought-provoking messages. We mailed them to every legislator at their homes in the summer and fall of 2003—before the legislative session was to begin in February, 2004.

"What if an automobile manufacturer produced millions of surplus cars each year only to have them senselessly destroyed? Would that make sense?" That was the message on the first card.

Card No. 2 read: "What if a company who manufactures computer components built millions of surplus parts each year and senselessly destroyed them all? Would that make sense?

"Can you as an intelligent human being think of any one thing that should be produced in excess by the millions each year only to be senselessly destroyed?" That was the message on Card No. 3.

The fourth week, the postcard read: "What is excessively produced in the State of Oklahoma each year by the millions and senselessly destroyed at taxpayer expense?"

OUR STRATEGY WAS to grab the short-spanned attention of most politicians by spoon-feeding them just a line or two of mysterious information. And it worked! A couple of our local representatives shared with us how the hot pink postcards had spiked their curiosity when they arrived in the mail at their homes each week for several weeks.

"What the hell is this about," one of them told me he was thinking when the cards would arrive. We hired former Senator Roy "Butch" Hooper to lobby for us. Butch was the senator who had spoken from the steps of the state capitol in the 1992 NOPO video, and was a believer in our cause. He convinced Lawton Senator Sam Helton to sponsor the bill.

I am certain I went through an entire ream of paper, appealing for financial help to every foundation in the State of Oklahoma, and beyond, that even hinted of an interest in animal issues. I think we may have received a total of $1,200 or $1,500.

Let's face it: We just have never been good at fund-raising. It seems that in this cause, you either spend a lot of time fund-raising or, in our case, you wing it and spend most of your time working hands-on with animals. It's a priority thing.

But then again, there's the foundation. That's the celebrity foundation in California set up to assist pet owners with neutering and spaying dogs across America. No one, anywhere, has been better to pet owners in Lawton and Southwest Oklahoma than this foundation. Over the years, it has provided the clinic with SNAP grants that have allowed us to neuter and spay pets for free or near free. In the eighth poorest state in the nation, that is phenomenal.

On more than one occasion, the generous foundation also replaced our worn out surgical equipment with what was called a "clinic grant." In 2012, I wrote a cover letter for our application for a clinic grant that began in the following manner: "Twenty seven years of operating a low-cost neuter/spay clinic in one of the poorest areas of the United States, takes a toll on volunteers, veterinarians, clinic staff and equipment. Realizing you can do nothing to help us with veterinarians, clinic staff and replacement of old worn out volunteers, we are, however, appealing to you once again to assist us in replacing well-worn surgery equipment and other needed items necessary to continue to provide high quality neuters and spays." Once again, the generous foundation came through for us with every needed piece of surgical equipment.

At the foundation's request, we have not been allowed to use the celebrity's name in press releases or advertisements about the monies. The grants, however, were discontinued—to all recipients—on July 31, 2014, and the story of these remarkable gifts could not possibly be absent from this book.

On each occasion of our requests to the California foundation, we invited the celebrity to our Lawton clinic to see what miracles his generosity has wrought. Fat chance. Didn't happen. But we tried.

WE CONTINUED TO send our hot pink postcards to the homes of legislators. The messages became more detailed: "A sign at Atwoods in Lawton advertises Great Dane mixed breed puppies for sale for $200," began one of the messages. "A sign next to it advertises a family garage sale. A nearby Pepsi machine has a $50 tax sticker attached. The garage sale requires a permit. But the dog owner and puppy vendor is not required to buy any permits to offer his product for sale. He should, by law, collect sales tax, but most don't! Tens of thousands of dogs and cats end up as strays on roads and in animal shelters and cost farmers, humane societies, and taxpayers millions. Breeding dogs and cats are Oklahoma vending machines. They should be taxed."

Another postcard read: "Want to start a business in Oklahoma? A restaurant maybe or a beauty salon or barber shop; perhaps a bowling alley or skating rink. A florist shop, or even a store that sells eggs. Get ready to buy lots of licenses and permits. Don't forget your state sales tax permit. And you'll pay toll fees if you must commute. But if you allow your dog or cat to have puppies or kittens and then sell or give them away . . . not to worry!!! No permits required! No fees required!! And if you don't find homes, (which you probably won't because there are tens of thousands of surplus ones born every day) you just take them to the country for the farmer to deal with. Or if you're halfway decent, you'll take them to the local animal shelter where Oklahomans spend $12,000,000 every year to kill them. Does this make sense?"

We had come up with the 12-million-dollar figure by way of calls to Oklahoma's largest communities. While I was begging foundations for grants, Linda was calling 20 municipally-operated shelters to inquire about their budgets. She faced a surprisingly large amount of resistance in her quest to obtain information from the larger shelters such as Oklahoma City and Tulsa. Tulsa, at the time, had a breeding law that was not enforced, however, it is my understanding the law is currently being enforced.

Interestingly enough, local sheriffs in smaller communities, who were providing animal control to their communities, were more receptive to laws that crack down on pet breeding than many of the staff of the larger shelters. Counties in Oklahoma do not have the luxury of animal control or animal shelters.

We had been talking about breeding laws almost since day one. We still are talking about it.

How anyone can work in this cause for two minutes without realizing you can't fix pet overpopulation with adoptions—or even neutering and spaying—is something I will never understand. It is amazing, however, how many humane societies and rescue organizations just don't get it.

Inasmuch as we were unable to obtain financial help from foundations, our lobbyist and our hot pink postcards were all we had. We could only hope that our legislators had been able to digest enough of our bite-sized, common-sense information to make a logical decision.

Oklahoma legislative attorneys drafted what became Senate Bill 1130, "The Dog and Cat Ownership Responsibility Act."

"For the purposes of this act," the bill read, 'Dog and Cat Ownership Responsibility' means responsible pet ownership by discouraging breeding, reducing pet over-population by encouraging spaying and neutering of pets, and ensuring that each cat and dog born in the State of Oklahoma has a good and permanent home."

Who could find fault with that? Well, other than dog and cat breeders; the American Kennel Club; an Oklahoma City TV personality; the executive assistant to Senator Helton, the bill's sponsor; Senator Nancy Riley of Tulsa who obviously resented everything about me and the bill; and...oh yes, the Oklahoma Veterinary Medical Association—to name just a few.

Barely was the ink dry on proposed Senate Bill 1130 when the proverbial excrement hit the fan. Before the legislative session even began, the AKC was prompting angry breeders and members to e-mail or call Oklahoma legislators to oppose the bill. This was not the AKC's first square dance; they had been busy stomping out these anti-breeding laws as they were cropping up across the country—and they were good at it! They still are!

The draft of the bill was dated January 21, 2004. By February 2, 2004, Lorettta R. Jones, executive assistant to Senator Helton, was sending an e-mail from "grapevine" to "Recipient list suppressed." I am certain we were never supposed to see that e-mail but someone on the "suppressed" list obviously forwarded the contents to Linda's e-mail. Jones listed the Subject as S.B. 1130 –"Cat and Dog" issue!! The message, which included multiple exclamation points, and capitalized letters for emphasis, read: "At the request of Senator Helton, S.B. 1130 (Cat & Dog bill) will NOT . . . (I repeat) . . . will NOT be heard this Session. Senator Helton didn't realize the complexity of this issue until after the Bill was filed. He wants to APOLOGIZE to all of you for the many calls and concerns this Bill has produced for each of you. Senator

Helton will NOT BRING BACK . . . S.B. 1130. THANK YOU for your understanding and patience during this ordeal!!!

This "ordeal" was a win-win situation for the State of Oklahoma. Pet owners would have been forced to take the responsible action of having their pets neutered or spayed, or purchase a license to do otherwise; and commercial breeders whose animals produce more than one litter per year would have been required to plunk down $1,000 for a license to breed multiple litters. This would have covered the state's hundreds of puppy mills.

Alcohol and tobacco carry hefty taxes in this country known as "sin" tax. Is there any greater sin perpetrated on American society than the overproduction of puppies and kittens that has resulted in the killing of billions of them over decades—at taxpayer expense?

Had this law passed, the State Department of Health would have contracted with motor license agents for the purpose of issuing licenses. When automobile owners renewed their car tag each year, they simply would renew their dog and cat licenses. Over time, Oklahoma citizens would have begun to realize it is unacceptable to not have their pets neutered and spayed.

The Oklahoma Veterinary Medical Association did their part in making sure the bill would be defeated. In the winter 2003 OVMA Legislative Report, written by Drs. Billy Clay and Russ Donathan, the OVMA makes clear veterinarians' opposition to the bill. "SB 1130 mandates spaying and neutering pets at an early age and imposes fees for Intact Licenses, Noncommercial Breeders Licenses and Commercial Breeder's Licenses. We, along with many others, have offered opposition to this Bill. The latest information is that it has been withdrawn but we will remain alert to its possible reappearance," the report read.

Yep! The Oklahoma Veterinary Medical Association was adamantly opposed to the "Oklahoma Dog and Cat Responsibility Act," right up there alongside breeders and the American Kennel Club.

Fully realizing I have posed the following question in this book multiple times, I, unashamedly, cannot resist asking it again: What is it that dead animals in landfills bring to veterinarians' practices that they have fought so hard for so long to preserve?

TV personality Kelly Ogle with KWTV in Oklahoma City editorialized against the bill in a segment entitled "My Two Cents." He ended his comments with the statement: "This dog won't hunt." When I called him to inquire as to why he was so opposed to the bill, he rudely implied that I was someone completely ignorant of the issues and asked me if I had "even read the law?"

Three years later I would have a more positive occasion on which to write a letter to Mr. Ogle.

None of this should have come as a surprise. Mark Harman, a savvy animal control officer from the small community of Bristow warned me. In a January 29, 2004, e-mail, he wrote that "you have climbed into a political arena wherein you will find the oppositions to be very mighty. As I am sure you know, should Oklahoma pass this bill they would be second to only New Hampshire. In any state, those in the business of ranching, agriculture and such will take such a proposed bill as a threat, fearing that its passage will open doors that they wish not to open."

I e-mailed Harman, after the bill failed, on January 31, 2004: "I agree with you that this kind of legislation is almost an impossibility in this state, but it was worth trying for as we believed if we pursued it from a taxpayer angle that perhaps we, by some miracle, could be successful. We made mistakes by not gathering support behind the scenes early on, but we were trying to be secretive about it to begin with and to tell you the truth, the way people are in this movement, I didn't know who to trust. Several "rescue" groups e-mailed against us.

"We have for sure been bloodied in this latest battle," I wrote to Harman. "I disagree with you only on one point in your message: that dog breeders love dogs. I can't comprehend how that could be possible knowing what happens in animal shelters day in . . . day out . . . year in . . . year out. When breeders produce litter after litter over and over and over again, knowing full well about pet overpopulation, I am hard pressed to believe that it is motivated by love for animals and not by money."

Both Harman and I shared the fact that each of us were ignorant regarding pet breeding early in our lives, and we agreed that we need massive public campaigns to reach others and prevent them from making the same mistakes.

"Chasing strays, sheltering them, loving them and then, yes, euthanizing them, has consumed us and we haven't had the time to fight the battle in the appropriate arenas," I wrote.

"We are not dead. We are just wounded. And we will continue to fight," I promised.

On January 30, 2004, I sent a letter to editor Ed Kelley at The Daily Oklahoman, Oklahoma's largest newspaper. Surprisingly, Mr. Kelley was kind enough to print a shortened version of the piece in a Sunday edition of his paper. *The Lawton Constitution* also printed my remarks.

"Taxpayers and animal welfare advocates took a bloody beating in the recent attempt at legislation to regulate pet breeding in the State of Oklahoma," I began.

"An excess of unwanted dogs and cats is a documented and escalating problem costing taxpayers billions over the years.

"Spewing the same old rhetoric and contrived propaganda, the pet breeding industry positioned proponents of the now defeated SB 1130 as extreme animal rights radicals hellbent on sweeping away their rights to own and breed purebred pets.

"Senator Sam Helton, who introduced the Oklahoma Dog and Cat Ownership Responsibility Act, succumbed under pressure from this special interest group, and supposedly from senate leadership, and dropped it like a hot potato.

"The breeders' modus operandi has always been to divert attention away from the indisputable facts: that pet breeding, whether it occurs in the family pet, a hobby breeder, or a puppy mill, contributes to overpopulation; and that the only hope we have of resolving this disgrace is to get a handle on the breeding that causes it, i.e. to a place where supply equals demand," I wrote.

"Make no mistake. This law would not have outlawed breeding. It's advocates were not PETA affiliates. It would simply have required breeders and irresponsible pet owners to pick up some of the $12 million tab borne by Oklahoma taxpayers to operate the killing houses we call animal shelters.

"Legislators have never been shy in imposing taxes and regulations. Considering the costs to taxpayers and society, it borders on insanity to allow this activity to continue to go unregulated."

"Breeders point to unaltered family pets and claim they are the only culprits," I pointed out. "But they refuse to look within their own ranks, including the infamous puppy mills for which this state is so well known, and admit their industry might actually benefit from sensible legislation.

"The basic rule of supply and demand is that you don't produce more of any product than you can sell or give away whether it be automobiles, computers, pogo sticks or dogs and cats. And if you do, it shouldn't become the responsibility of the taxpayer to deal with the excess.

"As long as pet owners fail to act responsibly and lawmakers fail to regulate responsibly, taxpayers will continue to lose. Individual rescuers, humane societies and shelter workers, who deal with the carnage on a daily basis, will continue to see little reason for hope.

"But the greatest losers are those who are senselessly destined for the euthanasia needle, or something far less humane. They die for a sin no greater than being born into a world where, because of politics and greed, supply far exceeds demand."

I ended the op-ed piece with a line I have been repeating for years.

"We are a civilized society. We can do better than this!"

Senator Nancy Riley of Tulsa scolded me severely in a letter that was not dated. She didn't like anything about the bill. The salutation was my first clue as to the angry tone of her letter. "Ms. Delluomo:" the letter began.

"I have received your pink postcards all interim. Two questions come to my mind: 1) Why didn't the person sending these postcards have the courage or integrity to put their name and address on the card? 2) Why are the messages so subliminal?

"I hope I have just received your final card blasting Senator Helton for "succumbing" to special interest groups. I know that Senator Helton was never contacted by the American Kennel Club. If his constituents were like mine, their outcry against this proposed legislation was overwhelming.

My email ran 10 - 1 AGAINST this bill. It seems that everywhere I went in my district, SB1130 was a topic of conversation and disbelief. I found *no one* in favor of this bill.

"Ms. Delluomo, I have no doubt that we need some action to curb the unwanted animal population in our state. However, your approach and tactics were not in the best interest of the average Oklahoma citizen. This was proven by the deluge of phone calls and emails that were received in every legislator's office voicing disapproval of SB1130.

"I strongly urge you to stop your personal vendetta against Senator Helton and learn how to achieve your goals in a more constructive, rational manner."

My feelings were hurt. But they've been hurt before. I ignored Senator Riley's letter—until a year or so later. On May 23, 2005, I responded. Excerpts from my letter to the senator reads as follows: "I am tardy in my reply to your less-than-cordial letter to me concerning the now very defunct SB1130, a bill that was and is so badly needed in the State of Oklahoma and around the nation. I had decided that your letter was not worthy of my response, but as I clean out my files and mentally revisit the issue, I have decided that I do have a few things to say to you.

"First, as expressed by the enraged tone of your letter, you exhibited a great dislike for me which I find disturbing in that you know nothing of my life's work and obviously you know even less about the pet overpopulation problem and how it is draining the lives and pocketbooks of so many good citizens of Oklahoma, many of whom are your constituents.

" . . . Because the AKC so readily mobilized their opposition to the bill and we who supported it were never given a chance to be heard, how could you possibly know if anyone supported the bill?

"You state in your letter that I blasted Senator Helton for succumbing to special interests. He did indeed do that. What kind of a person agrees to carry a bill and before a session even begins, toss it out before the proponents can be heard?

"And of course you were never contacted by the American Kennel Club. That would not be good strategy on their part, Ms. Riley. They instead had their breeder membership across the country flood you with e-mails and calls while we who supported the bill were overwhelmed and had been told by our lobbyist that it was too early to start to call legislators. It's tough, Ms. Riley, for citizens of one of the poorest states in the nation to compete with the rich and powerful American Kennel Club. If you think they were not behind the opposition, then you didn't check their website wherein they discussed defeating bills like it in other states.

"You posed two questions to me about the pink postcards sent to you 'all interim.' First, you ask why the person sending the cards didn't have the integrity and courage to sign his or her name; and why the messages were so subliminal.

"This, Ms. Riley, is called strategy. The withholding of my name was intentional in the early stages of that strategy in an effort to pique your interest. You notice names were affixed later into the effort.

"Surely, your friend Mr. Helton did tell you that I have been extremely dedicated and vocal (actually courageously vocal) on this subject for many years. And while I admit I have made enemies (mostly from those who have a vested interest in making sure there are never any regulations concerning the billion-dollar pet breeding industry, including many Oklahoma veterinarians), I have never been accused (except by you) of being too timid or too unethical to merely add my name to a postcard. To anyone who knows me, that is actually funny. So, Senator, you had it all wrong!

"Face it, Ms. Riley, you and every legislator in the state were duped by the AKC of New York City, and yet you take exception to my tactics and say they were not in the best interests of the citizens of Oklahoma. Unbelievable!

"As to your wish that you not receive any more "cards" from us, that is a commitment that I cannot make. While I realize that you personally are incapable of understanding the issue and choose only to see the personality aspects involved, I can tell you that I do understand it and I have been involved in the euthanasia of enough dogs and cats to cause me nightmares for the rest of my life. So, please understand, Ms. Riley, that as long as I have breath in me, I will continue to fight to end the senseless spending of taxpayers dollars on an impound and kill method of animal control. This battle is far from over...with or without your support.

"In closing, (if you're still reading this letter, which is doubtful since you didn't even want to be bothered to read a short message on a postcard), let me vehemently say that I do not have a personal vendetta against Mr. Helton as you erroneously charged. He agreed to carry a bill for a cause and dropped it as soon as the heat was turned up. That is an undebatable fact.

"And, once again on the subject of integrity, or perhaps just good manners, notice that I have begun my letter to you with a proper salutation, a courtesy I was not afforded in your letter to me.

"Perhaps, Senator Riley, instead of being so critical of someone you know absolutely nothing about, just perhaps, you should look at your own style of communication and professionalism . . . or the lack thereof."

I filed the letter in my computer under "Bitch Riley." OK. I admit it. That wasn't nice. But I never mailed the letter to Senator Riley; and my computer is private. And it did make me feel better, which I thought I deserved for spending so much time on a piece of legislation that went absolutely nowhere.

There was no doubt about it. Oklahoma was not ready for The Dog and Cat Ownership Responsibility Act. Obviously, neither is America!

CHAPTER 53

"I won't insult your intelligence by suggesting that you really believe what you just said." — William F. Buckley, Jr.

IN THE SPRING 2013 issue of its In Session newsletter, the AKC hypes its organization as the "Only not-for-profit purebred dog registry devoted to the health and well being of all dogs."

Seriously? Even all those millions of dogs, including purebreds, who die in animal shelters each year because of excessive pet breeding?

Was the "health and well being of all dogs" what the AKC was thinking when they lambasted Senate Bill 1130? Was the "health and well being of all dogs" in the collective conscience of the leadership of that organization when they were opposing the other hundreds, if not thousands, of pieces of legislation proposed by animal welfare advocates throughout the years.

The article claims they admonish breeders to "give careful consideration to health issues, temperament, and genetic screening as well as to careful placement of puppies in appropriate homes."

Really? Do the brass at the American Kennel Club in New York City truly believe that breeders, who sell puppies out of their garages and out of the back of pick up trucks and SUVs at Walmart, give a flip about whether the home is an appropriate one?

The AKC statement about "careful placement of puppies in appropriate homes" was made in the same breath in which they were murmuring their opposition to the Federal law that had just been passed to regulate Internet sales of puppies nationwide. Do the perpetrators of this propaganda want us to actually believe Internet puppy dealers have heretofore screened the purchasers of their commodities for appropriate homes any more assuredly than do back porch breeders who sell at flea markets and parking lots?

Make no mistake! It's all about the money. These small breeders pimp out their dogs for Christmas money in the winter and buy their kids' Easter outfits in the spring. Pet breeding, on the larger scale, is a billion-dollar industry.

Seriously, have the AKC suits ever set foot in a Midwestern puppy mill?

Is the AKC, as it proclaims, devoted to the health and well being of all dogs?

I don't think so!

But in the words of William F. Buckley, Jr. and as an act of kindness, I won't insult their intelligence by suggesting that they really believe what they just said.

CHAPTER 54

"If veterinarians weren't going to help the under served, then humane societies and rescue groups would fill the need. And today we see a proliferation of low-cost providers of veterinary services . . . The state veterinary boards started this problem. They can stop it by ending the harassment of veterinarians who want to provide low-cost services." — Gerald Dobesh, January 2015 issue of *DVM 360 magazine*

THE COVER STORY of the January 2015 issue of *DVM360 magazine* reads: "Low-cost; business-savvy. For-profit spay-neuter clinics seek to fill niche but battle resistance from veterinary colleagues."

Rachael Zimlich wrote that "the veterinary market has seen a blossoming of low-cost spay and neuter clinics as pet owners have struggled to pay for their pets' healthcare. Many are nonprofit programs that have drawn fire and even been challenged by law in some states. But for-profit spay and neuter clinics seek to find a middle ground—providing a reasonably priced service that provides enough revenue to support the business and its owner."

The article profiles several for-profit veterinarians who had ventured into the low-cost neuter and spay business. Interestingly enough, many of them have experienced the same resistance from veterinarians as we have experienced at the Animal Birth Control Clinic.

In the same issue of the trade publication for veterinarians, Gerald Dobesh, DVM, in a letter to the editor, blames the profession for non-profit spay clinics.

"Who caused the proliferation of low-cost spay clinics owned by charitable 501(c)3 organizations?," Dobesh asked.

The Omaha, Nebraska, veterinarian answered his own question. "We did," he wrote.

Dobesh stated in his letter that the problem for-profit veterinarians were encountering was state veterinary boards trying to shut down those who were already performing low-cost spays and neuters.

"Such veterinarians could count on fines, license restrictions, probation and other harassment from their state board. This created a shortage of low-cost providers that the low-income clients needed," wrote Dobesh.

Dobesh went on to explain that the profession began ignoring low-income clients and that opened the door to charitable organizations. "If veterinarians weren't going to help the under served, then humane societies and rescue groups would fill the need. And today we see a proliferation of low-cost providers of veterinary services.

"The state veterinary boards started this problem. They can stop it by ending the harassment of veterinarians who want to provide low-cost services. Low-cost clinics owned by veterinarians will charge higher prices than the 501(c)3 groups and at the same time outcompete them for business."

Now there's one of those few veterinarians who gets it—a veterinarian who has his head screwed on right.

I have my doubts, however, that the veterinary community will heed Dr. Dobesh's advice.

They didn't listen to the pleas of my hero, Dr. Lloyd Faulkner, when he said essentially the same thing forty-nine years ago in his article entitled "Spay Clinics." They have made sure to oppose breeding laws across the country. Is it any wonder I would have little faith that anything will be different going forward?

My pessimism was justified in 2015 when the City of Lawton hired G. Dale Fullerton, a rogue and corrupt investigator from the Oklahoma State Board of Veterinary Medical Examiners, to perform an investigation of serious wrongdoing and downright animal cruelty at the Lawton tax-supported animal shelter.

There can be no doubt about it. Years long vengeance against the Animal Birth Control Clinic played a significant role in the ultimate investigative report that would be provided to the City of Lawton by the OSBVME and their employee, G. Dale Fullerton.

CHAPTER 55

"I think controversy is not always a bad thing. Jesus was controversial. It's through controversy that people often wake up and smell the coffee and say, 'What's going on here? Do we need to rethink something here?'" — Kirk Cameron, Television Actor

A FEW DAYS ago I received a notice from the Oklahoma Tax Commission that the tag and registration on my car would be due for renewal in a couple of weeks and that I could either pay by mail or go to my local tag agency to take care of the charges. The notice also reminded me that I would need to provide insurance verification at the time of the renewal.

As I was driving to the tag agency, I was reminded of just how many rules and regulations apply when living in a civilized society. It occurred to me that registering my car and providing proof of insurance is not a whole lot different than registering or licensing animals with a municipality or state. We drive our cars on roads and highways built with tax dollars; and we must buy insurance, not necessarily to protect our vehicles, but to protect other drivers and passengers to which we might cause harm.

In 1993, I was invited by the Humane Society of Wichita Falls in Texas to be a guest speaker at a candlelight vigil for animals that had died in animal shelters. As I was rumbling through my old plastic tubs, I found a copy of the speech.

I spoke to the crowd about my hero, Dr. Lloyd Faulkner, who had written the article about veterinarian opposition to low-cost spay clinics back in 1971, and how 22 years later, at that time, little had changed. Now as I write this, 49 years after Dr. Faulkner wrote that article, I am devastated that once again I am lamenting that so little has changed in the cause for animals.

In that speech, I told the crowd that veterinarians had long been a tremendous stumbling block in the battle against pet overpopulation.

"There are others we can blame," I said. The list included pet pushers, pet shops, the AKC, the Department of Agriculture, unconcerned taxpayers who keep picking up the tab for animal control, medical technology for failing to give us more updated measures for pet sterilization.

"We can place blame until the cows come home," I said.

"But what about us. Where do we fit into the picture?" I asked.

"As we scrutinize the reasons we have never gotten from here to there, and we look at those people we've just talked about, we can at least see their reasons. They are indifferent, they are uninformed, they are in the game for money. So, from that standpoint, it's easy to see why the battle has not been won. Or, for that matter, why it's never even begun to be fought.

"But what's the matter with us, people?" I asked again. "What's the matter with us?

"We've known all along what the problem was. We didn't just get out of bed one morning and say, 'Damn, I know what causes all those dogs and cats and puppies and kittens at the animal shelter. It's pet breeding!! Why didn't I think of that before.

"But we kept telling ourselves we can adopt them out, or we'll get our literature in the schools and educate people, and we'll get some watered down licensing laws and we'll give away or subsidize neuters and spays . . . or better yet we'll take on the veterinarians and build our own neuter/spay clinics.

"We knew all along what the problem was. But we've been really busy. We've been really traveling along this road that for us has to be called 'Acceptance.' And you just can't get there from here on a road called 'Acceptance.'

"But like I said. We've been really busy. We've had to treat the mange and the distemper and the parvo and the broken bones of those who weren't quite street-smart enough.

"And we've been having to run our shelters and write our newsletters begging for money so we can continue to run our shelters and treat the mange and the distemper and the parvo and the broken bones. And we have to buy our traps to catch the ones who are out on the road and too frantic and too frightened to come to us and trust us to help them.

"And then we don't have any energy left or any money left to work for what's really needed to give us some rest. We can't drag ourselves to our city council meetings or our state legislatures to lobby for breeding laws or hire lobbyists to work for us.

"Do you know what would happen if we used just one-tenth of the money we spend to operate our shelters on lobbying our government for breeding laws? That's what the NRA does, it's what the AMA does, it's what the AKC does, it what the lawyers do, it's what the elderly do. It's what everybody does . . . but us!

"We've known all along what the problem was. But we've stayed quietly busy doing the dirty work. We've been loving them and holding them while we're putting a needle in their tiny veins and then tossing their limp bodies into a despicable heap . . . a heap just as dead and silent and despicable as our own reluctance to scream out against what we've known to be the problem all along. Pet breeding! All pet breeding!"

I ended my speech by imploring those in the crowd, who were each and every one a loving and compassionate individual, to rethink the way we do things in the world of animal welfare.

CHAPTER 56

"You're walking next to a river and you see a kitten floating past. You jump in and save the kitten. Then another one floats by, so you save that one, too. Then another and another and another float by, and you soon realize that you can't save them all. So you run upstream to see who's throwing kittens into the water—and you stop that person." — PETA

IF VETERINARIANS, THE State of Oklahoma and most of the rest of the nation were not ready for a "Dog and Cat Ownership Responsibility Act," the City of Lawton, now with an animal control budget up to half a million dollars, decided maybe it was time to go upstream and find out who was throwing kittens into the river.

On February 13, 2007, the Lawton City Council unanimously passed a tough, comprehensive anti-breeding law called the Breeding, Advertising and Transfer law or the BAT Permit law.

This law was patterned after the failed SB 1130 and not unlike the 1992 law that was passed but never once enforced due to politics and some veterinarian opposition. The animal control budget in 1992 was $250,000.

We fought hard to get the 1992 law enforced and, looking back, we should have brought legal action against the city. But there are just so many battles one can fight with a budget that will stretch only so far.

We, however, tried our best to get the law enforced. We purchased what was called the Jo-Jo television commercial that was being used in other states as a tool in getting breeding laws passed. The ad featured a beautiful Irish Setter who naively was unaware she was about to be euthanized. Accompanied by mournful background music, a male voice spoke: "This is Jo-Jo. All she ever wanted was a loving home. But Jo-Jo's world is coming to an end. Look away if you must, but know that this happens over and over every day in our community." Then, in all its emotionally anguishing reality, Jo-Jo's innocent life came to an abrupt end right before our very eyes in that thirty-second commercial. We added our tag at the end of the commercial asking citizens to support enforcement of the breeding ordinance to help end the killing insanity.

We didn't stop there. We ordered other literature. We distributed a four-page brochure which featured a beautiful puppy and kitten on the front with a caption which read: "Amy and Buster couldn't wait for the law to be enforced." On the center spread were photographs of Amy and Buster's lifeless bodies and the caption read: "Now they're dead!"

All this was to no avail. The law was never once enforced.

I HAVE MADE it abundantly clear in this book that throughout my animal activism, I have not endeared myself to many veterinarians, purebred dog fanciers, the American Kennel Club and a host of politicians—as well as some individuals in general. As I have stated earlier, it goes with the territory.

I will have to admit, however, that on the occasion of the passage of the BAT permit in Lawton, a law we had begged for and preached about for years, it was really amazing how the city council, the mayor, the city attorney, animal shelter personnel, the humane society and the Animal Birth Control Clinic came together to make the breeding law possible and perhaps one of the best in the nation.

ON APRIL 16, 2006, Linda and I placed a large ad in the local newspaper. The ad was entitled: "About cats and Laws . . . It's time to try new things. An Open Letter to the City of Lawton."

On April 23, 2006, we placed a second ad entitled, "About Cats, Dogs, and Laws . . . and Trying New Things."

What actually had prompted these ads was a law that had sneaked by us and passed by council at the urging of Rose Wilson, then Superintendent of Lawton Animal Welfare. We labeled it the starve the cats law. It was, sadly enough, still in force until recently, but most humane citizens continued to feed the cats which, historically, have been ignored by animal control.

I happened to be in Phoenix when Linda called to tell me about an article that appeared in the paper wherein an older Lawton couple had been assessed huge fines for placing cat food for homeless cats on their front porch, their own private property.

I responded with a letter to the editor. "As a sixty-eight-year-old woman who has spent most of my adult life fighting for the humane treatment of animals (including experiencing a politically motivated, crimeless arrest), I thought I had seen it all. And then an issue arises such as the one pertaining to the feeding of stray and starving animals and I find that I am sickened by the debate.

"Many decent people feed starving animals. Unlike animal control, they are not paid and often sacrifice to do so. The cats on the streets are there because for years animal control has not done its job pertaining to them. How difficult is that to conclude?

"Suffering is suffering and compassion is compassion," the letter continued. "And when we were told that when we do this, 'unto the least of these, we've done it unto Him,' I believe He meant all forms of life.

"Law or no law, if I encounter a hungry animal on the streets of Lawton or anywhere else for that matter, I will feed it as I have done my entire life. And I will risk arrest to do so. My spiritual welfare depends on it and my soul demands it."

Okay. I admit it. It is probably words such as the ones I wrote in the final paragraph of the letter that have gotten me in trouble from time to time over the years.

"I encourage other citizens to do the same. There is a higher calling within some, or even most of us, that will not be dictated to by an inhumane authority. It's called a conscience. And besides, what could be a higher, more moral form of civil disobedience!"

"YOU CAN'T SMOKE here. You can't smoke there. Fasten your seat belt. Get a garage sale permit. Buy a license if you want to hunt, fish, drive, cut hair, build or remodel houses, sell eggs, cigarettes, liquor, etc. 'Cosmetology fee hikes proposed' was a headline in this paper recently. Government is involved in almost every aspect of our lives."

That was the first paragraph of the newspaper ad we placed on April 23, 2006.

"Why in the name of heaven are lawmakers so reluctant to impose fees on the product of puppies and kittens, an activity that ultimately costs taxpayers millions over years and negatively impacts society in so many ways.

"Something is very wrong with a system that allows an activity that is so detrimental to society go unregulated, untaxed and uncontrolled," we wrote.

We asked the question: "Why do the wishes of those who profit from dogs and cats take precedent over society in general? Does anyone even consider the negative impact on those who work with the thousands of unwanted animals day after day after day? What about those who have to kill the unwanted thousands year after year? What about the good-hearted citizens who sacrifice to take in 'one more stray'?"

We pointed out in the ad that the animal control budget was now over half a million dollars and increasing every year.

Finally, we wrote; "We are at a crossroads. We can lag behind and be the last to take action. Or we can be innovative leaders and set the example."

SHORTLY AFTER THE ads ran in the newspaper, Linda received a strange, unexpected phone call. "What is it you all want?" asked the woman on the phone.

"Excuse me?" Linda responded.

"What is it you all want?" the woman repeated.

The woman on the phone was the founder of the now defunct Sheltering Tree Animal Rescue Society, an animal rescue organization she had formed in 2002 and run out of her tattoo and body piercing shop here in Lawton. Linda spoke to her a couple of times and had gone to one of her meetings when I was in Phoenix. We were always anxious to meet with and work with anyone truly advocating for the best interests of animals. We were, however, never clear on how she adopted out the large numbers of animals of which she claimed or just how her organization was run. We do know that she hauled animals around the country and that she and Rose Wilson were obviously good friends.

The woman explained to Linda that she was referring to our newspaper ads.

Linda explained that the starve the cats law had inspired us to place the ads. Starving animals to death is not the answer to pet overpopulation and neither is euthanizing. Linda told this woman, plain and simple, we want breeding laws! To this day, we still don't quite understand that call.

Ten months later, in February 2007, Lawton did set the example and passed the anti-breeding law, which might be, if dutifully enforced, one of the best in the nation. Its main drawback is that its boundaries only extend to the Lawton City limits and breeding continues throughout the county.

IMMEDIATELY, WE MAILED out press releases to virtually every news outlet in the State of Oklahoma touting this major innovative piece of legislation. We titled the press release Neuter, Spay or Pay.

"A litter of puppies or kittens born in Lawton could cost their owners a fine of $500 and a possible thirty-day sentence in the municipal jail."

That was the beginning sentence of the press release we provided to news media all across the State of Oklahoma.

"The Lawton City Council this week, in a unanimous vote, passed a groundbreaking "litter" ordinance that supporters say will provide relief for taxpayers and should be adopted statewide," the notice continued.

"Too many unwanted pets is always the most pressing problem facing animal control agencies," said Rose Wilson, Supervisor of Lawton's Animal Welfare Division, who drafted the law using the 2004 failed Oklahoma Senate Bill 1130, the "Dog and Cat Ownership Responsibility Act" as a partial guideline. "When pet owners refuse to have their pets neutered or spayed, taxpayers are impacted and animals die," she said.

"The Lawton ordinance penalizes pet owners who allow their animals to reproduce, whether accidentally or intentionally, by requiring them to purchase a Breeding, Advertising and Transfer (BAT) permit.

"The city requires one of two licenses, "A" or "B," for registration of animals. License "A" is for pets which have been spayed or neutered while "B" is for intact pets.

"A BAT permit allows the owner to breed only one litter per licensed animal per household per year and requires the permit number to be posted in any advertisement for puppies or kittens to be sold, given away, or transferred in any way. Should an animal accidentally breed, the owner must obtain a BAT permit immediately or submit the animal to be neutered or spayed.

"Kittens and puppies born in violation of the permit must be forfeited to the Animal Welfare Division and their owners are subject to a $500 fine or 30 days in jail, or both.

"The "B" license number must also be posted in pet stores on holding pens of animals offered for sale.

"A list of BAT permit holders will be provided by the City of Lawton at the end of each year to both the State and Federal Tax Commission.

"Wilson promises the law will be strictly enforced. 'I have good people at my shelter and, frankly, they are tired of killing healthy, beautiful pets,' she said.

"The Lawton based National Organization to End Pet Overpopulation has advocated this type legislation for two decades and were the initiators of SB 1130. "We pointed out to legislators in 2004 that just the major cities in Oklahoma spend well over $12 million each year to run shelters which often are little more than killing houses," said Linda Reinwand, NOPO treasurer. She said the state is also losing millions in tax revenues by not regulating pet breeding.

"To complicate the issue, there is no animal control in Oklahoma counties and rural residents must fend for themselves when faced with stray dogs and cats." said Reinwand.

"NOPO operates the Animal Birth Control Clinic, a low-cost, non-profit spay clinic in Lawton wherein at least 60 dogs and cats are neutered or spayed each week. Charitable grants ensure that no pet is turned away because of an owner's inability to pay.

"We're all set with a brand new $15,000 grant which means no pet owner needs to be impacted financially by this new law," said Deloris Delluomo, president of NOPO.

"Promoters of the ABC Clinic contend that their work of twenty-two years has greatly reduced the number of animal killings in Lawton but maintain the problem cannot be solved in any community that doesn't have mandatory neuter and spay laws.

"Our hats are off to our forward-thinking council members," Delluomo said. "I believe we can claim one of the best laws in the nation right here in Lawton and state legislators should definitely follow suit."

On February 14th I wrote a personal letter to Kelly Ogle of KWTV in Oklahoma City who had opposed SB1130 in his My Two Cents commentary back in 2004.

"Enclosed is a press release which has been sent to all media across the State of Oklahoma concerning an important ordinance passed Tuesday evening here in Lawton. The law seriously restricts the breeding of dogs and cats," I wrote.

"I wanted to be sure you received your own copy of this information because, if I recall correctly, you editorialized against the defeated SB 1130 initiated by our organization here in Lawton in 2004. Although I did not see your piece, I was told you ended it with, 'This dog won't hunt.' I also recall that you were rude on the phone implying I was someone completely ignorant of the issues when you asked if I had 'even read the law.'

"I assure you, Mr. Ogle, I am completely familiar with the horrors of pet overpopulation and I have been involved in the euthanasia of enough dogs and cats to cause me nightmares for the rest of my life. And I will continue to fight as long as I have breath within me to end the senseless spending of taxpayers dollars on an impound and kill method of animal control.

"What is so disturbing is how people such as yourself, blessed with a public forum, can give 'your two cents worth' about an issue you obviously have no experience in and know absolutely nothing about. How many animals have you held in your arms while they were being killed purely because no one anywhere wanted them or had room for them?

"Pet overpopulation has a tremendous negative impact on taxpayers and society as a whole, not to mention the suffering and deaths of millions of innocent pets. And it borders on insanity to allow the breeding of pets, whether accidentally or intentionally, to go unregulated! As you can readily see, our Lawton law is based partially on the 2004 proposed state law, but is even more comprehensive and restrictive. In other words, Mr. Ogle, in Lawton . . . This dog will hunt!"

I like to think I am a nice person, not given to gloating or bragging on occasions of a successful moment for the animal cause. But sometimes I just can't help myself!

ON FEBRUARY 23RD I wrote a letter to General David Ralston, Commander of the Fort Sill Military Base in which I requested his cooperation in applying the law to military residents at Fort Sill.

I explained to the commander that "Fort Sill pet owners account for many of our clients and we have sent neutered and spayed pets out into the world via those clients.

"Anything that you could do to partner with us in achieving our goals, such as assistance in creating an awareness of this law to military families, would be greatly appreciated," I wrote.

I closed the letter by expressing appreciation to him and the soldiers of Fort Sill and around the world for their service to our country.

I can't say whether or not any one at city hall heard from Fort Sill on this issue. I personally never had a response from General Ralston or anyone else at Fort Sill.

On February 16, 2007, I wrote to City Attorney John Vincent thanking him, his assistant attorney Frank Jenson, and his entire staff for the tremendous amount of work put forth on the newly adopted animal ordinances.

I told Vincent we were still not breathing easy considering what had happened to the same ordinance passed in 1992.

Unbelievably, one of the vocal opponents of the ordinance, a veterinarian, had told council on the night of the vote that "the numbers at the shelter have been the same for the past twenty years and that neutering and spaying has not been effective and is not the answer."

Millions and millions of dogs and cats without homes! That's called pet overpopulation! If humanely rendering those dogs and cats incapable of reproducing litters of puppies and kittens is not at least an absolutely vital part of the solution then what on God's earth does he suggest inasmuch as he was also against any anti-breeding or even licensing laws. This was the sort of nonsense with which we had been battling most local veterinarians for years.

In my letter, I set Attorney Vincent straight. I told him that we have information on a city letterhead that had been given to us by the former Animal Control Supervisor in the early 1980s when it was under the control of the police department. All the information I had saved from that time indicated that in the late eighties and early nineties, 7500 animals were being euthanized by the city.

I told Vincent that we had operated the shelter by contract for a bid, albeit totally inadequate, of $45,000 for the shelter part alone, and that the animal control budget was under $150,000 at that time and in 2007 was now well over the half-million-dollar mark and counting, but still inadequate for the current situation.

"As councilman Warren pointed out, the euthanasia figures for the past ten years has been consistent at 4500 to 5000," I wrote to Vincent.

"What we did not know in the beginning, but learned very quickly, is that the battle of overpopulation can never be won with only readily available and low-cost surgeries. We knew years ago it would take nothing short of laws that limit, tax and overall regulate pet breeding of all kind, accidental and purposeful, to end the insanity of killing as a means of animal control.

"With the death of that law back in 1992, we have never been able to get past that brick wall we hit at 4500 to 5000 animal shelter killings, a figure which only includes city shelter statistics, not ours from the ABC Clinic, not dead animals on the streets, not other veterinarians, and not animals dumped in the county," I wrote.

"Considering what happened in the past, we are, of course, concerned about some unforeseen "kink" in the enforcement of this law. Rumor is some of the naysayers are threatening legal action. Any such action would be a shame considering how meaningful this law can be to the welfare of this city if it is properly enforced.

I informed Vincent of the many phone calls we had received from throughout the state and beyond. I told him about the camera crew that had come to the clinic from OETA in Oklahoma City. I told him about the radio interview I had with Oklahoma News Service who asked if we wanted to make Lawton a model for other cities in Oklahoma with this law. "I told her for sure we do and that our ultimate goal is to be the first, not only in Oklahoma, but in the nation to boast a zero (0) euthanasia rate.

"With the current Miss America hailing from our city; Extreme Makeover Home Edition coming to town, and our expected influx of military families from other posts, this wonderful new animal "litter" ordinance is just one more instance of Lawton putting ourselves on the proverbial map.

I ended my letter to Vincent by profusely thanking him and his staff for the hard work on the ordinance and his ongoing service to the City of Lawton.

I also sent a letter to Deputy City Attorney Frank Jensen thanking him for "the long hours of time and labor that undoubtedly went into the drafting of this wonderful new ordinance . . . Please thank your assistants for their hard work and know that you are greatly appreciated."

I received a letter from Mr. Jensen dated February 22, 2007.

"Thank you for the kind words in your letter and recognition of the outstanding work of our assistants," Jenson wrote.

Obviously, Jensen was feeling somehow unsettled about possible legal ramifications due to the weigh-in of so many opponents, i.e. the special interest groups.

"In the event of litigation, I will be counting on your assistance with mounting a strong defense in support of the ordinance," he wrote.

One thing was certain. We had never seen in all our years of animal activism the kind of cooperation we had received from virtually every one at City Hall.

EVEN THOUGH THE anti-breeding law had support of virtually every branch of Lawton municipal government, it was not without its opponents. Not by a long shot!

Of course, the American Kennel Club had to weigh in on what was going on with dogs in Lawton, Oklahoma. On February 22, 2004, nine days after council unanimously passed the BAT Permit legislation, Walter R. Bebout, Director of Canine Legislation, wrote a letter to Mayor Purcell expressing his disapproval of our Animal Welfare ordinance No. 07-06 and "the method whereby the ordinance amendments were adopted with little public notice and limited opportunity for citizens of Lawton to have input into the process of amendment consideration.

"As a not-for-profit organization founded in 1884, the American Kennel Club (AKC) has been devoted to the advancement and welfare of dogs for 123 years. The AKC supports sound, enforceable, non-discriminatory legislation to govern dog ownership."

Bebout told the mayor that if "the goal of the Lawton City Council is to assure a high rate of compliance with an ordinance, then it is necessary to solicit public input in development of such an ordinance . . . For elected officials to truly represent their constituents, they must necessarily receive input from constituents. The extremely short timeframe (sic) between public notice of the animal welfare ordinance amendment consideration by the city council and final adoption did not allow the citizens of Lawton the opportunity for meaningful input regarding the amendment contents."

Bebout ended his letter by asking council to "reconsider the adoption of amendments to the animal welfare ordinance approved on February 13th, 2007, and that the effective date for the amended ordinance be postponed during council reconsideration of the ordinance amendments. The goal of reducing the number of unwanted dogs and cats is laudable but it is crucial that the right to own dogs and cats responsibly be protected in that process."

Duh! I could be wrong, but . . . no . . . no. I'm quite sure that the purpose of the ordinance in the first place was for citizens to own dogs and cats responsibly.

What the hell was Mr. Walter R. Bebout of the American Kennel Club talking about? The BAT Permit law that was passed in Lawton, Oklahoma, on February 14, 2007, was fiercely debated, talked about, argued about and written about. Breeders, dog show advocates, some veterinarians, the sports editor of the daily newspaper and any other opponents were anything but silent.

We had experienced the bully behavior of the American Kennel Club in a big way in 2004 in Oklahoma City at the state level. They were trying to do it to us again here in Lawton. Somehow, they had missed the mark and failed to rev up the pre-emptive propaganda machine in time to flood city leaders with opposition letters before the council vote as they had done against SB 1130 in 2004. Now they were asking that the ordinance be put on hold until they could get the propaganda machine up and running. We were wet behind the ears in the state arena of politics, but we knew our way around city hall and how to mobilize support for animals in Lawton. We were not going to lose to the intimidations of the powerful giant again.

On February 23, 2007, I wrote a letter to Mayor John Purcell letting him know we had heard about the letter from the American Kennel Club and their opposition to the "litter" ordinance.

"The AKC is a wealthy organization, headquartered in New York City," I wrote. I explained to the mayor that they register hundreds of thousands of dogs from the infamous puppy mills in this state, and they have done little or nothing to address the deplorable conditions in which most of these animals spend their lives.

I told Mayor Purcell that it was imperative for council members and staff to understand that any influx of e-mails opposing the ordinance might be coming from AKC members across the nation, not necessarily Lawton citizens.

I informed Mayor Purcell that the Animal Birth Control Clinic had been inundated with calls from citizens who want to comply with the ordinance and assured him there was statewide interest in the law.

"There is no doubt that Rose Wilson and her Lawton staff, not the American Kennel Club of New York City, are the best judges of what this city needs to address the overproduction of unwanted dogs and cats," I wrote.

"In closing, a pertinent thought comes to mind: Since the American Kennel Club is so concerned with dogs and the governmental affairs of the City of Lawton, perhaps its highly paid directors should come to Lawton and comfort the animals at the city shelter as they are administered the needle of death on euthanasia day," I suggested at the end of the letter.

ON THE EVENING the law was passed, a huge crowd of supporters were walking out of the council auditorium alongside breeders and other opponents of the law.

"I hope you're happy," some person I had never met said to me as we walked outside the council chambers. "You just took away my ability to make a living."

"Why don't you get a job for yourself instead of your dog."

That was how I so desperately wanted to respond. I, however, didn't say a word. I just kept walking. Hopefully, God gave me a couple of points for that one.

This dog breeder was not the only one who was unhappy with our new ground-breaking, life-saving animal ordinance. Pet shops, dog show fanciers and breeders were waking up to just how they perceived their own bottom lines would be impacted by this new law. And even disgruntled citizens, i.e. pet owners, good ole boys in general were deciding that no one has the right to tell them what they can or cannot do with their "damn dogs." Joe Kiehn, veterinarian and former council member, was telling council and anyone who would listen that neutering and spaying had not affected the numbers of animals killed at the animal shelter.

On February 18, 2007, I sent a letter to the editor about the lies that were being perpetuated by Dr. Kiehn and others.

"I am becoming weary (if not downright angry) about the erroneous information being put out that the numbers at the animal shelter have been the same for the past twenty years and that neutering and spaying has not been effective and is not the answer," I wrote.

"Nothing could be farther from the truth!"

"Perhaps Dr. Joe Kiehn's memory needs to be refreshed," I wrote.

I once again explained what the euthanasia numbers were when we started the neuter/spay work and how they had been cut in half.

"What some may not know is we had a law such as this new one back in 1992. Joe Kiehn and his ilk, i.e. breeders, pet shops and those whose interest lies in money for themselves and not in the interest of taxpayers, animals and the community overall were successful in getting the law shot down. We can only pray that this doesn't happen again," I wrote.

"My question to Joe Kiehn and his cohorts is this" If pet breeding doesn't cause pet overpopulation, please tell me what does. Duh! I don't think he knows the answer.

"The city council, I believe, spoke for the vast majority of decent citizens on February 13th by voting unanimously for this breeding ordinance. No decent person in his right mind can believe that killing is an acceptable manner by which to curb a pet overpopulation problem.

"You can educate children all you want, neuter and spay until you are blue in the face, try to convince those who already have too many animals to adopt one more, blame this pet owner or that one, but until pet breeding is taxed and regulated, the slaughter of innocent pets will continue at an ever-increasing cost to taxpayers. Supply must equal demand. End of argument!"

On February 26, 2007, Linda sent out an e-mail urgent message, the subject being "New Animal Ordinances."

"Just wanted to let you know that the breeders have been hard at work to overturn the new ordinances. The mayor was sent a letter from the AKC (dogs' worst enemy), with copies to the city council members and Lawton Dog Fanciers stating the public did not have a chance to let their objections be heard . . . It has been wild at the clinic all week. It is amazing how many people have decided they need to have their purebred dogs neutered all at once. We are booking into April and will get into May next week. We are working on a surgical team coming to Lawton to perform extra surgeries on a Friday and Saturday. We will be receiving a grant from the Kirkpatrick Family Fund in Oklahoma City for neutering/spaying cats. Your continued support will be greatly appreciated."

On March 22, 2007, Linda sent out another e-mail to supporters asking once again for support to keep the ordinance intact.

"Here we go again," she wrote. After our great victory for the animals at the city council's meeting on 2-13, new councilman Jim Hanna is going to put it on the agenda at the 3-27 meeting to put it on hold, and for a committee to study the ordinances.

"This is exactly what has happened in the past, and they form 'stacked' committees made up of breeders, pet store owners, Dog Fanciers, and some vets (only a couple really are against the ordinances . . . Joe Kiehn and Scott Briggs. They promise to 'committee' the ordinances to death," Linda wrote.

"We are doing a mailing to all citizens in Lawton who have signed our petition at the clinic but we need everyone to try to get as many people at the council meeting at 6:00 at City Hall on 3-27! Please be there and bring as many people as you can. We can't do it without your help. The opposition has had time to get organized, and these ordinances have to have a chance to work.

"I can tell you that we have been overwhelmed at the clinic with neuters/spays (many, many purebred large dogs), and many full-term pregnant dogs which have all been large dogs. These pet owners have put their animals at risk all for money! They just could not be bothered until they realized they would not be able to sell the puppies without the BAT permit. The other truly amazing thing is the amount of vaccinations we are doing. People have been in violation of state law by not even having their animals vaccinated for rabies! We are seeing six and seven-year-old dogs to be neutered or spayed and receive their first vaccinations. Many, many of the dogs are purebreds and are covered in ticks and fleas. These are the so called 'responsible' pet owners. Once again, please come and bring many, many people with you. An hour of your time for the animals is time well spent."

On Tuesday, March 13, 2007, Joey Goodman, a sports writer for *the Lawton Constitution*, in the sports section of all places, voiced his strong opposition to the ordinance and his obvious hatred of me. Several people called to tell me about the scathing article, one of whom was Councilman Keith Jackson. A photo of a chain link fence gate at the animal shelter with a sign on it that said "closed" accompanied the article. Goodman was angry that when he went to the shelter to purchase a license for his puppy he found the "gates padlocked. Yes, you read that right," he wrote, "a government office complex locked on a Monday. And to make matters worse, it's just two days before this wide-ranging ordinance takes effect." Goodman obviously was unaware that the shelter closed on Monday because it was open on Saturdays to accomodate citizens on their days off.

"You know the ordinance I'm talking about, the one that was shoved down our City Council's throats by one woman who obviously has time to hound lawmakers instead of making a living like the rest of us middle-class Lawtonians.

"It's an ordinance that most all of the veterinarians this writer knows says won't work in cutting down on the number of animals that are running free on the streets. What it will cause is more and more helpless animals being dumped in the country, and believe you me, having grown up in the country, I know about having things dumped on our rural roads.

"Obviously the City Council just got tired of hearing this woman hounding them and voted for this policy just to get her out of their hair. Well, I think there are going to be a good many Lawtonians go to the City Council meeting tonight to voice their disapproval and they won't be ones who have been coached about what to say by the woman in question.

"No, these are going to be law-abiding citizens who are tired of things like this happening and having them forced down their throats.

"Let me tell you about this woman. It used to be she called to complain to this desk every time we'd run a picture of a hunter with a trophy mount, or whenever we'd run a story about the rodeo. She hates hunting and she hates rodeo and she wants both to be eliminated.

"If I want to hunt or go to a rodeo, then I should have that right and I think there are a bunch of people like me and I hope they attend the Council meeting tonight and voice their objections.

Goodman finished his rant about me with his own suggestions about letting veterinarians and pet shops and groomers sell dog and cat city licenses. He suggested that perhaps if the City Council "won't roll back this huge ordinance totally, maybe they will put it on hold for sixty days and put together a panel of veterinarians, business owners and common pet owners to look at ideas that will develop a simpler ordinance that will make sense . . ."

I had never met or set eyes on this man, Joey Goodman. I had never even heard of him. I don't read sports sections of newspapers. Almost everything he wrote was out of ignorance about the ordinance, and what he wrote about me were outright lies. I went to the newspaper and demanded space to set the record straight. Considering what probably was the libelous nature of Goodman's rant about me, the newspaper allowed me to counter Goodman's misguided knowledge of the ordinance and his knowledge, or lack thereof, of me personally. I labeled the piece "An Open Letter to Joey Goodman."

"No one ever said life would be fair," I began my rebuttal. "That point was once again driven home by you, Mr. Goodman, in your column of March 13th.

"While I overwhelmingly defend your right to disagree with our new Lawton animal ordinance and even my political tactics, I do, however, have a huge problem with personal attacks. That's well below the belt.

"Could you provide me with dates when I supposedly contacted your "desk" to complain about any article in the sports section, be it rodeo, hunting or otherwise? That wouldn't be my style. If I have something to say about an article in your newspaper, I write a letter to the editor as is the proper etiquette.

"To the best of my knowledge, I have never spoken to you in my entire life. I can count on one hand the number of times I have opened up the sports section of any newspaper.

"Forgive me, Mr. Goodman, but I don't even know who you are. So imagine my surprise when I received a call on the morning of March 13th informing me about your "sports" column, in which you describe your perception of my philosophies on rodeo and hunting, i.e. 'she hates hunting and she also hates rodeo . . .'

"While I admit, I am not a fan of hunting or rodeos (I have a problem with the broken necks of baby calves in roping events), in years past my late husband provided Nissan pickups to the LO Ranger rodeos and my son unloaded the barrels for the barrel racing event. My husband was an advertiser and a supporter of that event throughout the years.

"You seem to depict me as a woman of privilege, as one who has never known hard work and has only time on my hands to 'hound' City Council members.

"Actually, you and I do have some things in common. It might interest you to know that I, too, was raised in the country. I was born in a family of cattle ranchers and farmers, and curiously enough, hunters, in the Elgin community and you might also be surprised to learn that my mother and I milked cows by hand which we bottled and sold in the Elgin community to pay the doctor bills for my ailing father who died when I was thirteen.

"Yes, Mr. Goodman, I am an Okie through and through. I know about being poor. I know about hard work. And I know about hunting and rodeos, and eliminating them is not on my agenda. Not by a long shot!

"What I am about is ending the animal cruelty at our own back door; the one we as a society have come to accept; the one where we senselessly kill thousands of excess dogs and cats at a cost of millions to taxpayers and we don't even blink an eye! And if laws to address that cruelty inconvenience or displease you and a handful of breeders or veterinarians, then it is a small price to pay to end this ongoing insanity.

"You mention the amount of type that it took to print the ordinance in your paper, but are you aware of the months and months of intensive thought and labor that went into the drafting of this ordinance? Not by me, mind you but by Rose Wilson, Supervisor of Lawton's Animal Welfare Division, and by the City Attorney's office. Ms. Wilson was most likely working on those ordinances on Monday, one of her days off in that her 'government office complex' is open on Saturdays to better accommodate Lawton citizens.

"Wouldn't common sense dictate that Ms. Wilson, in light of her very job title is in the best position to know the needs of Lawton when it comes to animal laws? Her department does handle some 7500 dogs and cats each year and they see more instances of animal cruelties caused by pet overpopulation than you would probably even want to know about.

"Have you given any thought to the city employees who have to kill these healthy, beautiful animals each and every work day? Are you aware that workers quit their jobs because they just can't take it any longer?

"Recently, I was taken to task by a sensitive animal control officer for using the word "kill" in something I had written about pet overpopulation. What he doesn't understand is that I am personally tired of assuaging the conscience of an indifferent or uninformed public with softened terms such as "euthanasia" or "putting them to sleep."

"Before you became so critical of this ordinance did it ever occur to you what it does to a person mentally who rescues animals from near death and after a period of time of bonding, has no alternative but to kill them becaue there is just no where to put them?

"Do you even begin to understand the seriousness of pet overpopulation on individual lives; of those who can't bring themselves to terms with the killing and, therefore, wind up in the poor house because they become overwhelmed with more pets than they can ever feed or care for? We see them all the time at the Animal Birth Control Clinic.

"Many of these people then become labeled "hoarders" or animal "collectors"and the next thing you know someone is having to rescue the animals from the rescuers . . . usually with television cameras rolling.

"Do you know that in just the larger communities of Oklahoma, taxpayers shell out over $12,000,000 each and every year to run the killing houses we call animal shelters?

"Has it ever occurred to you that because there is virtually no animal control in Oklahoma counties, farmers and ranchers are left to fend for themselves and often lose cattle and sheep to a pack of stray dogs trying to survive? I know many of those farmers and, believe it or not, they support these laws.

"Do you really think Oklahoma's infamous puppy mills do anything to boost the image of the State of Oklahoma? Are you aware that in California there is a saying that "Oklahoma has the dumbest people and the most dogs" because of those puppy mills. Are you comfortable with that image of our state? I'm not!

"Should I continue on, Mr. Goodman? Because I haven't even scratched the surface of the far-reaching negative ramifications that the over production of dogs and cats has on society.

"Surely you know that in Oklahoma every business and activity is regulated or requires permits or licenses or is taxed in some manner. Can you help me in your column one day to understand why pet breeders, who inflict so much damage on society are, and should continue to be, allowed to walk away scot free?

"Did it not occur to you that it is because I have lived most of my life in the country and been forced to deal with an unending supply of dogs and cats dumped on my doorstep, that I ever became involved in this struggle against pet overpopulation in the first place? It's not something I do for fun!

"There has been a mentality for years, and for the most part, still exists, that pet adoptions can end pet overpopulation; that homes can be found for them all; or that if we just educate school children, as breeders and the American Kennel Club contend, we can end this merciless and senseless killing.

"And then we have the frantic neutering and spaying efforts in which we offer low-cost or no-cost surgeries. Would you be surprised to know that even when we make appointments at the Animal Birth Control Clinic for give-away surgeries, oftentimes these pet owners can't be bothered to even show up? What do we do about these people, Mr. Goodman, if we can't penalize them for being irresponsible and dumping litters of puppies and kittens on society when they have been offered options? Is this not where ordinances and laws become necessary?

"Over the years, humane societies and animal welfare advocates have been really good housekeepers for the breeders and other irresponsible pet owners in our society. We've cleaned up after them, and been damned quiet about it while we swept the dirty little killing secrets under the rug. That's no longer going to happen! We're shouting it from the rooftops!

"The latest is that the newly-elected Councilman Hanna is going to try to bring this ordinance back onto the agenda for reconsideration and there is at least one council person who is waffling. Those of us who have worked so very hard for so many years to address this tragedy of pet overpopulation are once again seeing our efforts undermined and this wonderful new law in jeopardy.

"You, Mr. Goodman, have something wonderful that is not available to me and others; and that is a public forum. I am asking you to search your heart, and your common sense, and find out exactly what this new law is supposed to do. And then, hopefully, you would use that forum to give this desperately needed law your overwhelming support!"

AS LATE AS July, 29, 2007, more than five months after the ordinance was passed, an ad that claimed to be paid for by "The Citizens of Lawton, OK" appeared in the local paper with a headline that read: LAWTON UNDER SIEGE BY THE ANIMAL RIGHTS MOVEMENT. It contained the usual tired old breeder-speak rhetoric: "They have taken away our rights to own unaltered animals without paying high fees...Do we want to live in fear of owning animals in the future? We do live in America, but it doesn't seem like that in Lawton . . . The ordinance is only the beginning as the activist (sic) take small segments of our animal rights away. Just small steps, but at the end we lose all."

The next to last paragraph of the ad was an interesting one. It would perhaps provide some insight into the actions of Councilman Keith Jackson eight years later. "City councilman Keith Jackson of ward 4 has voted in favor of the activist (sic) at each meeting. Do you want someone with such a liberal voting record to go on to represent our state in the future. A (sic) Animal Rights Movement Activist Representative in office at the state level is VERY SCARY. It starts with dogs and cats, but where do they stop? THEY DON'T."

Long time Dog Fancier Club member Billye McNeil wrote a letter to the editor asking how far were the city council, mayor, city manager and the city attorney going to go "in controlling our civil liberties? The animal rights movement is exploiting animal lovers around the world by using half-truths and scare tactics to push their hidden agenda. These groups campaign for animal rights, which is not synonymous with animal welfare . . ." wrote McNeil.

On March 19, 2007, Councilman Jackson forwarded an e-mail to Linda from a Mark Edwards on the subject of "HONESTY." The message was all in caps with dozens of exclamations points after every sentence.

"DID THE MAYOR TELL YOU ABOUT THIS!!!!!!!!!! THIS HAS BEEN FORWARDED TO NEWSPAPER AND TV STATIONS YOU HAD YOUR CHANCE TO BE HONEST BUT NOW THE PEOPLE WILL KNOW HOW DECEITFUL YOU REALLY ARE!!!!!!!!AKC APPEAL IGNORED BY MAYOR.

The angry sender of the e-mail message to Jackson included a copy of the letter from the AKC which was sent to the mayor "which he has refused to answer or publicly acknowledge!!!!!!"

ANIMAL RIGHTS MOVEMENT HAS LAWTON UNDER SIEGE. That was the headline of another ad placed in the local paper on August 5, 2007, five months after the BAT Permit breeding law was passed. The ad claimed to be paid for by the Citizens of Lawton and C.E. Ball, Blanchard, OK. "What will you lose?" the ad asked. "1. Privacy Rights; 2. Personal Property Rights; 3. Civil Rights." What will they lose? NOTHING!!!!!!!The ad continued on and on and on about all the rights of pet owners and breeders.

On June 7, 2007, A Whippet breeder named Walt e-mailed Shelly, neither of whom I know, wherein I was lambasted for the Lawton law. "This is a small community but the resident that pushes this craziness has pull with the council due to land opportunities and finances. She also has national affiliations. She was behind a piece of statewide msn legislation two years ago that was shot down. Let's see, would that be Delorus (sic) Delluomo?"

The e-mail claimed we were somehow rich and privileged and associated with an animal rights movement that was happening throughout the nation.

"If they can't get it done at the state level, they work covertly one community at a time with people who are embedded in communities and have clout with decision makers. And it appears the strategy is to target communities where that (sic) are naive, and have little contact with larger more metro parts of the state. That seems to be the plan here in OK," Walt wrote.

Walt told his friend that we "target all communities and states. In some places where their leadership is particularly strong, they have wealthy and well connected allies (newspaper may be bought), local pet lovers are naive and don't get (or reject) outside help, they succeed. Every combination that you can imagine has occurred regularly." The writing continued on for another page and a half, but it was completely clear that Walt the Whippet breeder had a fear and hatred of the animal welfare (or in his words AR community).

Shelly responded to Walt's e-mail on June 18, 2007. "Thank you for your insight! I hope you don't mind but I shared your posted response with my local dog club, members of the Lawton dog club and the OK pet law list serve."

I found the next paragraph of Shelly's response unsettling. In fact, it was almost frightening.

She wrote to Walt: "Thank you for responding. With the information you provided I hope to raise the level of concern that this is a small community but is one battle that must be fought. I think the fact that someone from outside the state recognized an ar person from 'lil ole Lawton OK' demonstrates that she is a serious threat and needs to be neutralized."

I don't have a clue what "needs to be neutralized" implies, but just to be safe, I took the correspondence to the Oklahoma State Bureau of Investigation where I knew a couple of agents and jokingly told them to keep it just in case "something happens to me."

Oh, that we had the clout, the money, and the organization with which these screaming angry breeders were crediting us. Do these same people purchase angry ads aimed at their state government and tag agencies for forcing them to register, tag, and purchase insurance for their automobiles? Dogs and cats and automobiles are considered personal property and both require millions of tax dollars for roads and animal control agencies. What's the difference?

They both should be regulated!

CHAPTER 57

"My father taught me many things here—he taught me in this room. He taught me—keep your friends close but your enemies closer." — Michael Corleone in T*he Godfather Part II* By Mario Puzo and Francis Ford Coppola

AFTER HOURS AND hours of debate about the new Bat Permit anti-breeding ordinance among pet shops, breeders, the AKC, the dog fanciers, and hate groups in general, and dozens of newspaper articles on the subject, the Bat Permit remained law in Lawton. And, as far as we knew, it was being enforced by the Lawton Animal Welfare Division. Because of the new law and the fact that it was being enforced, and our faith that the animal shelter was in relatively good hands, one might say we were living in what perhaps could be called animal welfare bliss. It wouldn't take long, however, for us to learn that our faith in a well-run animal shelter could only ultimately be described as ignorant bliss.

IT'S DIFFICULT TO describe my bygone relationship with the now former supervisor of the City of Lawton's Animal Welfare Division for more than two decades. It certainly never reached the trust levels of a friendship. There were no lunches, no meetings after work for cocktails. A business relationship? Perhaps. It most likely was an unwritten mutual understanding between the two of us. Something perhaps akin to a quid pro quo.

"Deloris, you and Rose have to get along," City Attorney Frank Jensen had said to me a few years ago. I had called Jensen about a problem we were having getting Rose to act on what we deemed to be an abandonment and cruelty case. A small dog had been left in an empty house in freezing temperatures. A couple next door to the house had become frustrated in their attempts to get help for the dog from animal control, and had come to the clinic to ask if there was anything we could do. In spite of the presence of a local humane society, which we had founded back in 1986, we still seemed to be the "go-to" place when citizens were frustrated with the Animal Welfare Division.

Rose insisted she knew the owners of the dog and that it was being fed. Pascall and Susan insisted on seeing for themselves. On arriving at the vacant house, they were able to see the small dog in a large window on the front porch. It wasn't difficult to see that the dog's water was frozen in the bowl.

Rose's refusal to take action left us no recourse. She was invoking the tired, old universal animal control excuse for inaction—that legally there was nothing she could do. I called Jensen. He did indeed agree with me that it was a case of abandonment, but at the end of the conversation, he admonished me to "get along" with Rose. I suppose his thinking was that Rose was in a position of governmental authority and I had long been a citizen with a loud voice for animals and, therefore, it was better for us to get along than to clash.

I'm not sure whatever happened to that little dog. I know it was eventually moved out of that empty house, due to our urging, but I fear it remained with its same owners.

Linda says with tongue-in-cheek that "the devil you know is better than the one you don't," so, throughout the years, we made every attempt to get along with the woman in charge at the Lawton Animal Shelter.

And we had, after all, in that letter back in 1987 to City Manager Melissa Vossmer, promised that we would always have an interest in a humanely-run animal shelter. "This decision (to not renew our contract with the city to operate the shelter) by no means indicates that we have lost interest in the shelter and the welfare of the animals there," the letter stated. "On the contrary, in our role as protectors of animal welfare, we will continue to have a serious interest in the activities of the shelter, regardless of who operates it after us, as it is, after all, the largest focus of animal-related activity and hands-on involvement within the community."

Surprisingly, Rose and I had the same philosophy on many aspects of animal welfare. Or, at least, I thought we did. That was perhaps the glue that held our curious relationship together. We emphatically agreed that the no-kill movement will never solve the pet overpopulation problem.

Until recent years, Rose's animal control officers had been at the clinic on a fairly regular basis delivering adopted animals for neutering or spaying, in compliance with Oklahoma law. Pascall and Susan actually became friends with a couple of them. But sometime around 2013, perhaps because of an incident involving the clinic and an emaciated pit bull, Rose began distancing herself and the shelter from the clinic. Dr. Haney, who had headed up the Animal Advisory Committee during the two-year stint when the for-profit Lawton Animal League operated the shelter in the late eighties, has been the shelter veterinarian since.

According to Rose, Dr. Haney was, at that time, performing neuter/spay surgeries in a closet at the shelter. That is, until Lawton citizens voted for what they believed, due to the wording of the proposition, would be a badly-needed new shelter for the animals, but turned out instead to be new offices for Rose and her staff and a new surgery unit for Dr. Haney. Lawton citizens were not happy when they learned they had been duped.

As it turned out, the dog kennels had little or no heat in the winter, injured dogs languished for days in pain with no medical care, no bedding was provided even though it had been donated, and nutritious and palatable food was non-existent.

Needless to say, Linda nor I knew just how bad the situation was deteriorating at the shelter. We desperately wanted to believe she was doing a good job.

She had, after all, along with Lawton City attorneys, especially Jensen, worked hard drafting the mandatory neuter/spay law for which we had lobbied for years. The language of the law, for the most part, was taken directly from the failed 2004 SB1130. Once passed, we made sure we gave credit where credit was due, and purchased an ad in the local newspaper thanking Rose, as well as all Lawton officials, for supporting the law. Also at the time, we were convinced that Rose was doing a good job of enforcing the law.

It was Rose who had called me in 2014 regarding the failure of the Fort Sill veterinarian and stray facility to adhere to Lawton's neuter/spay law, nor to the Oklahoma Dog and Cat Sterilization act, because it made their adoptions cheaper. In her position, it was most likely difficult for her to criticize anything regarding the military post.

Rose had done me a personal favor in 2008 by calling Dr. Silva at Animal Care and Control in Phoenix in an effort to assist us in bringing Pumpkin back to Oklahoma; and in late 2013 when I had a run-in with an arrogant Oklahoma City animal control officer over two small dogs that had been abandoned in an apartment there, she intervened on my behalf.

We helped Rose on multiple other occasions. Her officers had confiscated five Boxer puppies being offered for sale in the Walmart parking lot by breeders from the nearby rural community of Walters. This was a violation of the neuter/spay law, however, Rose was taking a lot of heat from Councilman Keith Jackson, who was advocating for the breeders and proposing that the City return the puppies to their owners.

As far as we could tell, Rose had handled the situation according to the law. She had confiscated the puppies, and had them adopted by city employees very quickly. The owners of the Boxers were demanding the city pay them $2500 for the puppies, and rumor had it that council was considering doing just that.

On the evening the council was to vote on whether or not to pay the puppy breeders, we attended the meeting and implored the council to not make that mistake.

"We are requesting . . . that the claim of $2500 for five boxer puppies be denied on several grounds," I told council members. I suggested if they agreed to pay for the puppies, they would indeed be opening a Pandora's box.

"First of all, I said, "How is it possible to determine the value of the puppies? And if you pay for these puppies, what's to keep the owners of the countless other puppies that have been confiscated from demanding payment in amounts that would be impossible to verify?"

I reminded council that animal control acted exactly in accordance with the law that was written by city attorneys, voted on and passed in 2007.

Council voted against paying for the Boxer puppies. They did, however, unwisely vote to revise the law which would allow owners of puppies or kittens confiscated under the Bat Permit, to pay their fines and be allowed to retrieve their breeding commodities.

On another occasion, Linda had read in the newspaper that an item had been placed on the council agenda to vote on transferring funds from some of the divisions' accounts. One of these accounts was designated by Oklahoma law to be set up specifically for unclaimed neuter/spay deposits and to be used only for programs that promote surgical neutering and spaying. We approached council who were mainly unaware of the law surrounding the account and it was saved for Rose's neuter/spay work at the shelter. We would deeply regret our intervention a couple of years later when we learned dogs had died from use of the chemical, calcium chloride, an experimental method of neutering male dogs which was being used at the shelter.

To sum it up, our relationship with Rose was a mixed bag. She had authority over the animal shelter, animal control and all things animal with the City of Lawton. Overall, it's not hard, then, to recognize that we did need to have some sort of a semi-cordial working relationship with Rose. But to say that we ever felt comfortable that all was well at the animal shelter would be a blatant lie. The tell tale signs were all around us.

It was 2012 and I had just walked into the clinic.

Susan grabbed my attention and asked me to follow her back to the dog kennels.

"Deloris, I want you to look at this dog," she said.

A low level of anxiety came over me as I sensed the urgency in Susan's voice and I was dreading what I might be seeing.

When we reached the kennel room, we stopped in front of the four-by-eight-foot tiled kennel which housed a white male pit bull. Although the dog had the distinctive large stature of the pit bull breed, it was one of the most emaciated dogs I had ever seen.

I had a million questions. "Where did this dog come from? Why is it here? Surely we're not going to neuter it in that condition, are we?"

"It was impounded by animal control," Susan revealed. "And, yes, it was brought here to be neutered but the doctor said he won't neuter it until it gains some weight."

Susan explained that animal control had impounded the dog a couple of weeks before. When she had quizzed the officer whether or not he had written the owner a ticket for neglect or abuse, he told her that it wasn't in that condition when they got it.

"Is the dog sick," I asked. "Will it not eat?"

"No," Susan answered. "He eats like crazy. We just got him yesterday and I think he has already gained a pound. "They also had him listed and housed as a dangerous dog, but he is one of the most loveable dogs I have ever seen."

I learned the dog's name was Kilo and when I reached down to pat him, he indeed seemed to relish the attention.

To say I was livid is an understatement. "This dog is not going back to that shelter," I said emphatically. "Do you hear me, Susan? If they try to come and take the dog back, you call me. I will go to jail, but this dog is not going back to that shelter!"

Once again, I was putting myself in jeopardy. The dog had been impounded by the City of Lawton and they would have had every right to demand the dog back. But I had already experienced a few hours in jail. How much worse could it get? And the dog was worth the risk!

That, however, didn't happen.

I made a phone call to Rose Wilson.

"Rose, what's the deal with the pit bull?" I asked.

"Well, Deloris," she snapped. "I guess he just doesn't like the food we have down here." That came as no surprise. It was no secret that shelter animals were fed the cheapest quality of food that could be purchased. The reason was always blamed on budgetary concerns in spite of the fact that the ever-ballooning budget was now up to three-quarters of a million dollars. But what we didn't know at the time was that the food budget was being depleted by Rose's bizarre personal hobby of maintaining what equated to a "zoo," and a poorly run one at that, at the tax-supported animal shelter, complete with everything from llamas to lizards, peacocks, emus, alpacas, ferrets, spiders, and a gigantic "tortoise in a box." And that is an incomplete list.

At that time, I couldn't understand Rose's response. Rather than assuring me she would get to the bottom of why Kilo had gotten into that condition, she was angry with me! If an employee at the Animal Birth Control Clinic had neglected an animal under our care in such a reckless manner, they would have, without a doubt, been fired.

Rumors would later circulate that dogs deemed dangerous breeds were routinely not fed as they were destined for euthanasia. I have no way to confirm that allegation, however, considering what would be revealed in later weeks concerning shelter policies, I wouldn't be surprised.

This incident with Kilo was too serious to ignore.

The next day, on June 14, 2012, I composed a letter to Rose from both Linda, who serves as director of the ABC Clinic, and I. The letter read as follows:

"On June 13, 2012, Officer Roy Roderick with the Lawton Animal Welfare Division brought a white male Pit Bull to the Animal Birth Control Clinic to be neutered.

"The dog was in an obvious emaciated condition and stressed with kennel cough. When a veterinary assistant inquired as to whether the owner had been cited for animal abuse or neglect, she was told by Officer Roderick that the dog was not in that condition when it was brought into the Lawton Animal Shelter two weeks ago.

"Dr. William Barrett refused to perform the requested neuter surgery due to the dog's poor condition and advised that the dog should remain at the clinic until his condition improves and the facts surrounding the issue could be sorted out.

"We were advised when the dog came in that it had been held at the animal shelter as a vicious dog. However, it was immediately obvious that this was not the case. To the contrary, this dog is very gentle and loving and interacts in a friendly manner with both humans and other animals at the Animal Birth Control Clinic.

"Dr. Barrett has placed the dog on an antibiotic for the kennel cough and has prescribed vitamins and a nutritional diet and the dog has responded beautifully.

"It should be noted that it is a violation of the Oklahoma Veterinary Practice Act to fail to report to the proper authorities cruel or negligent treatment of an animal by any person when the veterinarian has direct knowledge of such treatment.

"Inasmuch as this negligence occurred while the dog was in the care and custody of the Lawton Animal Welfare Division, we are at a loss to know just who the proper authorities would be. We wish to make it perfectly clear that we do not know every detail or fact in this case. We only can verify the emaciated condition of the dog on its arrival at the Animal Birth Control Clinic and are extremely concerned that this could have happened without being noticed and reported by an animal shelter employee.

"If this animal, or any animal, being held at the Lawton Animal Welfare Division refuses to eat the food provided and is noticeably losing weight, perhaps there should be a reevaluation of the sort of nutrition being fed to the animals.

"Let us not forget that for many of these animals, these meals will most likely be their last. Can we not as citizens and taxpayers afford to, at the very least, provide palatable food before they are euthanized?

"What is also disconcerting is the fact that this sweet, gentle dog was treated as a vicious animal, and most likely handled accordingly, during his stay at the Lawton Animal Shelter.

"We can only hope that this incident will provide a wake-up call to those who are charged with the care of these animals on a daily basis."

Copies of the letter went to the mayor, the city manager, the city attorney, every council member, and some members of the media. Channel 7 news picked up the story and questioned Jerry Ihler, head of Public Works, the division under which the animal shelter operated, who again blamed budgetary matters for unpalatable food and, more or less, said nothing could be done. Animal control claimed they were investigating the "allegations" and had contacted the Oklahoma State Board of Veterinary Medical Examiners to look at the case and would give an answer to our letter to city council that same week.

We received no response whatsoever from any city official or the Oklahoma State Board of Veterinary Medical Examiners on this incident. Not one. Nothing! Nada! Zilch!

I DON'T BELIEVE I spoke to Jerry Ihler, Rose's supervisor, about the pit bull incident. In fact, I don't recall ever having met, nor even spoken to him until late in 2014, when a kennel worker at the shelter wrote and distributed to council a scathing analysis of inhumane conditions in his workplace, a copy of which reached the Animal Birth Control Clinic. We would learn that at least one dog had starved to death and several others had died of complications of calcium chloride castration (an experimental neutering procedure of which Lawtonians had no knowledge). We would also later learn that more than 200 dogs and cats were found dead in their cages in 2013, which is the equivalent of one every other day. That number came from the department's own records under a column labeled DIP for dead in pen. When we operated the animal shelter back in 1986, we didn't even have a DIP column in our records.

Soon, after the kennel worker's letter was distributed to council, to the humane society, to us at the clinic, and reportedly to veterinarians, a fullblown tsunami of citizen complaints would flood across the Facebook landscape, exposing an inhumanely-run, tax-supported shelter that seemed to be right back where it was in 1986, or worse, forcing us to realize just how naive and inattentive we had actually been to conditions that had been developing there for years while we had been living in the trusting comfort of our ignorant bliss.

In December 2014, 18 months after the Kilo incident and the death of a dog from starvation was blamed on budgetary concerns, Rose Wilson would move into her shiny new offices and Haney into his surgical unit which, according to a newspaper report written by Kim McConnell, had cost Lawton taxpayers $662,000. Rose told McConnell that she did, in the future, plan to improve the building that houses the animals which would include installing a "new ventilation system to help control a majority of the problems (such as kennel cough) that plague the shelter."

In March 2015, after the release to the public of a libelous investigative report by G. Dale Fullerton, an employee of the Oklahoma State Board of Veterinary Medical Examiners, which mainly blamed citizens for all the problems at the Lawton Animal Shelter, Jerry Ihler would be promoted to city manager; Rose Wilson would no longer have her position as shelter supervisor, but would remain on the city's payroll, out of sight, at the library; and the two whistle blower kennel workers would no longer have their jobs with the City of Lawton.

In his contemptuous report, G. Dale Fullerton listed Linda and I, along with Susan, Pascall, Beverly Perry, Linda Wilson, Cathy Aycock, Renee Turner, whistle blowers Eric Stavinoha and David Nelson, and kennel worker Kenneth Dixon, along with our phone numbers and social security numbers which he then provided to the council and local district attorney requesting criminal charges be brought against us—for exercising our First Amendment rights!

The absence of honesty in this "hatchet job" of a report defies even an ounce of credibility or morality! So why did the City of Lawton allow it to ever be released to the public? Who were they protecting? And why?

CHAPTER 58

"When the axe entered the forest, the trees said, "Look, the handle is one of us!" — Turkish Proverb

MY RELATIONSHIP WITH Keith Jackson goes back more than 30 years— the entire duration of my involvement with the animal cause in Lawton.

I had thought of him as a friend. If that had actually been true, then I might never have been entering his place of business on that Thursday morning in March 2015, carrying a cumbersome 464-page investigative report of the Lawton Animal Shelter.

As I had quickly scanned over the index at City Hall, I immediately knew this report was what one local attorney would later refer to as a "hatchet job." And I was one of the trees.

When the City had called on the Oklahoma State Board of Veterinary Medical Examiners to handle the investigation, I expected a report that would attempt to malign the Animal Birth Control Clinic if for no other reason than the fact that the Federal Trade Commission had ruled against them 26 years earlier with regard to the legality of a low-cost neuter/spay clinic.

I had immediately shared that concern with Keith. He had called to inform me that the City was going to bring in someone to look at the allegations of mismanagement and inhumane treatment of animals that were being levied against animal shelter management. I recall, in that conversation, that he was less than transparent about who it was that had been called.

"Is it someone or some agency who cities call on to investigate trouble in certain divisions?" I asked. I knew there were professional shelter services who do that sort of troubleshooting for municipalities because we had called on a couple when we operated the shelter back in the eighties.

"Yes," it's an agency like that," he had said. He purposefully hadn't told me who the agency was in that he knew perfectly well about the history of the Clinic and the OSBVME.

Later on that day, I would learn it was indeed the OSBVME who had been called. I was outraged. I knew the investigator had a serious conflict of interest and I made sure I let Keith know. Not only was the OSBVME the agency who had harassed veterinarians at the Animal Birth Control Clinic for years, but it would turn out the investigator was a friend of Ruth Steinberger, the woman who had introduced the experimental calcium chloride neutering of male dogs to the Lawton Animal Shelter until it was halted by the city manager after citizens learned of its use, and that there had been serious unreported complications and deaths of multiple dogs.

Ruth Steinberger was also a lifetime Honorary member of the Oklahoma Veterinary Medical Association.

And if that wasn't enough of a conflict of interest, it would later be revealed that Rose Wilson herself had been allowed to choose who she wanted to investigate her shelter. Then there was Dr. Haney who had never been a friend of the Animal Birth Control Clinic, all of which begs the question: Who were the real conspirators in the investigation at the Lawton Animal Shelter?

Even knowing firsthand of the history between the Clinic and the OSBVME, and that Fullerton had those multiple conflicts of interest, I could not have imagined the report he would write (if he was even the one who wrote it) would have been so shamelessly dishonest and morally corrupt.

THE JACKSON LAUNDROMAT is a small "mom and pop" operation. As I entered the building and made my way through a row of washing machines, Keith saw me from his position behind a Formica-covered counter.

There was no doubt. He knew why I was there.

I walked up to the counter and slammed the report down right in front of him. Frankly, I don't remember exactly what I said, but I am sure it was language of which I might later regret. But then again, probably not! The tears rolling down my cheeks were not just a result of shock and hurt feelings. I was mad. I was raging mad. How could he have done this to me? How could he and his buddies at City Hall have done this to all of us?

And the greater and lingering question was: Why?

In a cold, smug manner, which frankly was unfamiliar to me as far as Keith was concerned, the Lawton city councilman took the report from my hands, opened it to the first page right after the index and, without saying a word, pointed to the heading at the top of a diagram which read "Conspiracy and Connection of Defendants."

Somehow, I had missed this all-important page while thumbing through the report at City Hall.

My angst began rising to a new level.

At the very bottom of the page was another connection in the diagram. It was a description of the overall conspiracy theory of G. Dale Fullerton, the investigator for the Oklahoma State Board of Veterinary Medical Examiners.

Fullerton wrote that the defendants had "Met on or about January 10 or 11, 2015 (his uncertainty of the date was typical of the mistakes, innuendoes and outright lies within the report) and conspired with ABC Clinic, the LCHTA and the members of Complaints and Concerns about the Lawton Animal Shelter Facebook Group (created by Susan Barmettler) to damage Lawton Animal Welfare and its employees and to set forth the events as outlined in this report."

I was listed as one of the "defendants." So was Linda, Susan, Pascall and Renee Turner (who is not associated with the ABC Clinic). Beverly Perry, who had created the Lawton Citizens for the Humane Treatment of Animals Facebook (LCHTA) page, was also listed, along with her mother, Linda Wilson, and her sister, Cathy Aycock.

A box in the middle of the diagram connected us at the ABC Clinic with Perry, Wilson, and Aycock, labeling us "Close Personal Friends," even though some of us had only recently met.

The kennel worker, i.e. whistle blower, who had written the letter of discontent with Rose and conditions at the animal shelter and sent it to all council members, as well as another worker who had also complained, were also listed as "defendants."

Actual charges that Fullerton had requested be filed against us had been withheld from his report and it would be three years (after a lawsuit was filed) before any of us would have a clue as to what charges the investigator recommended be brought against us. No charges have ever been filed and considering the ridiculousness of the charges, we don't expect they ever will.

Keith has been on the Lawton City Council for more years than I can recall. He represented Ward Four twice and now represents Ward Two.

The general consensus about Keith seems to be that he is politically ambitious. He has won seats on the council those multiple times, although he lost his bid for state office on two occasions.

A few years ago, I would have unequivocally described him as a friend and someone who had at least some heart for animals and that he believed what we were advocating was good for the City of Lawton. In spite of what happened in the animal shelter investigation, and his role in protecting the wrongdoing while maligning compassionate citizens, I will always be grateful for the multiple times he did vote responsibly in favor of Lawton's animals and taxpaying citizens.

He had asked me to write campaign materials for him in his bids for city office. In the last election for the council seat, his wife called me the night he was elected. In her excitement, she showered me with praise for my part in writing the material. In a brochure he had asked me to write, he promised to "hold the line against runaway spending and utility hikes." Lawton historically balances its budget on water rate hikes and Keith championed the most recent one in spite of his campaign promise.

Keith has passionately wanted to get to the State Legislature. That may provide a window into why he took the stand he did regarding the shelter investigation. Word on the street was that he felt he may have lost his first attempt at the state level because of his support for the Bat Permit.

Putting together the ads that the opponents of the law had taken out in 2007 about Lawton being under siege and mentioning him as a supporter of what they called the animal rights movement, and a letter I found in my old plastic tubs of ofttimes painful memories, it could have possibly played a role in his negative attitude toward us in 2015 with regard to the shelter investigation and his upcoming bid for the State Legislature. We may never know for sure.

In those old plastic tubs, I found a letter I wrote to Keith dated January 25, 2007, a month before the Bat Permit was passed which indicated we were not sure we would be able to count on his support for the law.

Excerpts from that letter are as follows: "As you are aware, we have fought for some sort of law for years to deal with the ever increasing animal control expenditures in this city. When Rose drafted this law, we thought for sure you were the one we could count on; that you for sure had an astute comprehension of the problems and the need for sensible solutions . . .

"We have never approached you and others asking for larger budgets for animal welfare. We haven't asked for a better building or better food for the animals. We advocate not larger shelters, but empty shelters which would free up tax dollars to be utilized in ways far superior to impounding and killing unwanted dogs and cats.

"How is it that you can repeatedly place surcharges on and raise the water rates which affect the poor and elderly, yet you express concern for those who are too lazy or irresponsible merely to have their pets neutered or spayed, which is the only means by which we will ever solve our ever-ongoing animal problems.

"You might be surprised to know, as we ourselves were indeed surprised to discover, that of the five other council members that we have had the opportunity to speak to thus far, you are the only one who has expressed reservations or fear of political fallout. In fact, Bob Shanklin met us that same afternoon at our clinic and told us he saw no problem whatsoever with the ordinance and didn't feel the licenses were excessive. He also went so far as to sign our petition at the clinic supporting mandatory neuter/spay laws in Lawton.

"So you can imagine our frustration and disappointment at your reluctance and negativity about this much-needed law which we feel is supported by so many good citizens, by the supervisor of the animal shelter and, we believe, even by City Hall.

"With regard to your comment about citizens just "wanting to be left alone," I think we all understand that concept but, in reality, most of us are willing to do what we must in order to fit into a civilized society. Whether we like to admit it or not, our actions do impact others and nowhere is this more evident than in the area of irresponsible pet ownership.

"On the attached pages, I have listed some pertinent examples of how government, including local, state and federal, hardly "leave people alone." And for the life of me, I can't understand your position in supporting this premise when it comes to the problems of an oversupply of unwanted dogs and cats and the hundreds of thousands of tax dollars required to deal with them.

"In closing, let me say that it would be wonderful if you could come to the conclusion that what we are advocating here, based on years and years of experience, is the right thing to do and that ultimately you would vote for it, not grudgingly because you feel pressured, but based on your gut conviction that it is truly in the best interests of the majority of the citizens of Lawton. Anything short of that will not be the long overdue and true victory we seek."

I added a P.S. to the letter: "Keith, if you genuinely think this will hurt your political career, maybe you should just not vote for the ordinance. I would hate to think if you lost the election, you would blame this one ordinance. I truly think we have the votes without yours, but it would have been so wonderful if we had a unanimous vote. We already have A and B licenses now and some people do and some don't comply. That doesn't concern me. What does concern me is that they have litters of puppies and kittens and the negative impact that has on all of us. (People take litters of puppies and kittens to the shelter hauling them in gunny sacks or sit on Sheridan Road outside Walmart giving them away or selling them. Is this the City we want? The only time those people who don't buy general licenses will be penalized is if their dog or cat gets impounded by animal control or has a litter of puppies or kittens. This is truly a near perfect law!

I added an attachment to the letter listing twelve instances of citizens who might want to be "left alone."

I spoke about our taxes and how most of us would prefer to be "left alone" when it is time to pay our Federal, State and local property taxes.

"Most people who have garage sales would probably prefer not to have to go down to get a permit and then pay taxes on their sales," I wrote.

"Those who hunt or fish would probably not like to have to go buy more than one license to be able to enjoy that activity.

"Those who enjoy the lakes with their boats probably would prefer not to have to buy a license to be able to put their boat in the water.

"I personally don't like to wear my seat belt and feel that I don't harm anyone else by not doing so, yet it is the law that I 'buckle up.'

"Those who operate vending machines probably would like to not be required to place stickers from the OTC on their machines and just 'be left alone,' but it's the law.

"From personal experience, I had to have a sales person's license when my husband had a car dealership to legally be able to drive a "demo" or car off of our own car lot. But that was the case and once I got stopped by a trooper who inquired of me, 'what authority do you have to be driving a car with a dealer tag?'

"Probably every dealership, store, restaurant and business service imaginable would prefer not to have to obtain the multiple permits and licenses they are required to carry.

"I suppose smokers really want "to be left alone" to smoke wherever they please. But their smoke impacts on the rest of us so we have laws restricting their activity.

"When we purchase tires, we pay a tax on our old tires because they have to be disposed of in public landfills. What about the 5,000 or so dogs and cats that go to the landfill each and every year to decompose in the ground? Where are the taxes for the people who once owned those animals?

"Yesterday, at our clinic, Linda and I were trying to take some of the clutter that had amassed off the walls, i.e. product information, notices, hours of operation, etc. When I started to take down some notices from OSHA, the Wage and Hour Board, and others, Linda reprimanded me and told me we must display those by law. Shoot, I didn't like the way they look. I wish we could have been "left alone."

"In the case of farmers, often they are told what crops they can and cannot plant. Betcha they'd like to be "left alone."

"Actually, there are hundreds upon hundreds of activities and businesses in Oklahoma which require permits and licenses as pointed out in a newspaper article several years ago. I don't have time to sit here and list them nor do you have time to read them. But, hopefully, you get my drift!

"Please vote for the ordinance that will require a segment of the population that causes so much harm to taxpayers, individuals and communities to put a "sticker" on their puppies and kittens because they are indeed "Oklahoma vending machines."

Keith did ultimately vote for the Bat Permit, along with every other council member. Whether or not he lost the state election due to that vote will probably never be known.

I HAVE ALREADY written that the report released on March 19, 2015, by G. Dale Fullerton and the OSBVME, and ultimately by the City of Lawton, was full of statements taken out of context, innuendoes, half-truths, and downright lies—mostly the latter. To try to make heads nor tails of the incorrect and deceitful information within the report is an absolute impossibility.

The fact that a dog starved to death at the animal shelter—let me repeat that—a dog starved to death!—or that more than 200 dogs and cats were found dead in their cages in 2014 did not appear to concern the investigator or very few others at City Hall.

What did indeed irk them was the creation of two Facebook sites, wherein almost 2,000 members contributed their experiences and their concerns of wrongdoing and inhumane treatment of animals at the animal shelter, however, the investigator, for the most part, ignored—if not ridiculed—the sincere complaints of concerned taxpaying citizens.

Fullerton and his cohorts, Shelter Supervisor Rose Wilson, calcium chloride advocate Ruth Steinberger, Dr. Howard Haney, a longtime opponent of the Animal Birth Control Clinic and the veterinarian performing the experimental calcium chloride neutering of male dogs, and the investigator of the OSBVME had their own agendas.

Fullerton had wanted to meet with Linda and I, and Pascall and Susan very early on and we initially agreed. However, in that Beverly Perry and General Baxter (Ret.) had, more or less, taken over the process of gathering information from citizens at the request of the mayor, we decided it was best not to meet with him. I spoke to Fullerton only once, I believe, perhaps twice, and I recall in that first conversation, he told me that he already knew that "charges would be filed" as a result of the investigation. He told others that also. I foolishly believed it would be animal cruelty charges against people at the animal shelter. How could I ever have known he would press for charges to be filed against those of us who asked that the animal shelter be investigated!

A section of the report entitled "CHARGES" was withheld from the report that was released to the public. This was the section that Fullerton took to the local district attorney's office requesting criminal charges (misdemeanors and felonies) be brought against those of us at the ABC Clinic and anyone who dared to be associated with us or criticize the animal shelter. We have only recently learned what was in those charges as it was released through the discovery process of a lawsuit being brought against Fullerton by Beverly Perry and her mother, Linda Wilson, two of the citizens who were severely maligned in the report. Perry had created one of the Facebook pages called Lawton Citizens for the Humane Treatment of Animals (LCHTA), and drew the wrath of the investigator mostly due to what he incorrectly believed to be her relationship to the Animal Birth Control Clinic, and the fact that the mayor had asked her to collect citizen complaints and report them.

The first paragraph of the "CHARGES" are indicative of the vitriol of the overall report that maligns citizens and protects city employees to the extent of promoting one of them to the position of city manager: "In that Deloris Delluomo and Linda Reinwand conspired (Title 21, Section 421) with their employees at ABC Clinic Pascall Osborne and Susan Barmettler and at the time LAW kennel employees David Nelson and Erik Stavinoha, along with Beverly Perry, Cathrin Aycock and Linda Wilson. At the direction of Delluomo and Reinwand the Facebook page of Complaints and Concerns about the Lawton Animal Shelter was created. Then the ABC Clinic employees joined forces with Beverly Perry and the LCHTA members and the kennel employees Nelson and Stavinoha. The above mentioned defendants used a computer network (Facebook) and devised a scheme to defraud, deceive and extort for the purpose of controlling the LAW, mayor, city manager, and city council. This scheme was designed from the onset for ABC Clinic to do all the spays and neuters for the City of Lawton and for retribution against Rose Wilson and Ruth Steinberger for not mentioning ABC Clinic in the writing and news articles. As a crowd sourcer Beverly Perry enlisted her mother Linda Wilson and sister Cathy Aycock to assist with this artifice by promoting mistruths and false information. In turn Beverly Perry's profession as a crowd sourcer would receive publicity in violation of (Computer Crimes Act) Title 21 § 1953 A2 and is a felony."

And that was just the first of the 16 charges Fullerton asked to be filed against us.

The question remains: What happened to Keith Jackson after all those years of supporting a humanly-run animal shelter? Where was his voice for the truth? What happened to Dr. Rosemary Bellino, who leaked out the whistle blower's letter to the president of the humane society, Phyllis Robertson, who then distributed it to us and others, and was the catalyst that, more or less, brought on the investigation? Fullerton was heard to say that Robertson was a wonderful person.

Could it be that she escaped his wrath because she was not associated with the Animal Birth Control Clinic? Dr. Bellino was my daughter's personal physician during her struggle with cancer, and she had told me in a phone conversation at the beginning of the shelter fiasco that she thought Rose "had to go." I had shared with her that I was so sorry this trouble at the shelter was being discovered and that my involvement would be minimal as my daughter was my first priority. On an occasion when Dana was in the hospital, as her cancer progressed, there were multiple times when Dr. Bellino could have mentioned the shelter report and at least told me she didn't believe we had done any of what the investigator had accused us of—twice when we were in the elevator together and other times in Dana's room. And, after all, she had told Dana when I was living in Phoenix before Dana's cancer was discovered that "Lawton was a better place when your mother was here." Where was her voice for what she had to know was the truth?

And then what about the other six council members? They had to know, given our lengthy past history of animal activism carried out with integrity, that none of us had committed any crimes in speaking out against an inhumanely run, tax-supported animal shelter? Why did they approve the release of this libelous report which will remain on the internet throughout eternity?

I HAVE SPENT thirty-five years of my life attempting to make this a more humane community. And it's not just for animals. When someone has called for help, it has never been an animal on the phone. It is always a person needing help. Many years ago, a Fletcher resident found a stray dog. She called whoever was in charge there and they told her to call the Comanche County Sheriff, who, in turn, told her to call Dan Delluomo Nissan and provided the number to the dealership. I, of course, went to Fletcher and got the dog. It was common practice for someone needing help with an animal to call Dan Delluomo Nissan. People who I don't know have approached me in Walmart to say "thank you" for something that happened years ago. Several months ago, a woman was in the clinic and as I came in the door, she stopped me and told me how much the clinic had helped her.

"I get strays dumped on me all the time and without this clinic, I couldn't have made it," she said. We hear that from people all the time.

Linda and I have not just talked the talk. We have walked the walk. As the saying goes, we have put our time and money where our mouths were. In 1991,when we were still in charge of the humane society, during a six-month period we picked up eighty-one dogs and cats in the county at the request of the sheriff and were never compensated in any manner—nor ever even thanked.

I have not even mentioned in this book about the cattle and horse cruelty cases we were involved in and that Dan and I kept many of those animals at our home. In fact, Sheriff Kenny Stradley adopted two Paso Fino horses that had been confiscated in a cruelty case.

Linda went through an agonizing time when her twin sister, Sharon, was dying of leukemia. Linda was donating her stem cells and spending hours, days and weeks by her sister's side, but she managed to make sure the administrative work at the clinic wasn't neglected.

Whether they would ever admit it or not, the City of Lawton has benefitted tremendously from the availability of low-cost (or no cost) neuters and spays in this community. It has saved the city multiple tax dollars and lessened the number of animals handled at the shelter. Historically, pet owners who have used the clinic would not have been able to afford a full-service veterinarian.

For the City of Lawton to allow Fullerton's report to be made public was mind-boggling and hurtful for Linda and I who felt we had given so much. It was weeks before we could speak of it without being brought to tears. Given our history, however, it was what we would have expected from the OSBVME.

One thing for sure is that we have never been accused of starving a dog to death; nor refusing pain medicine for animals in pain; nor finding dead animals in our kennels every other day. It's always been about the animals for us. Yes, we've been vocal and we've fought hard, but we've done it with integrity–in spite of what G. Dale Fullerton and the OSBVME would have anyone believe.

For years, I have had this silly saying. It is totally grammatically incorrect and it goes like this:"I got a Humanitarian of the Year Award from the Humane Society of Wichita Falls (Texas); I got a letter of commendation from Patrick Parkes of the Humane Society of the United States for the Animal Birth Control Clinic and my battle against pet overpopulation; I got a write-up in the Doris Day Animal League Magazine after the rescue of the twenty-eight bird dogs from Norman; and in Lawton—I got arrested!

MY BELOVED DAUGHTER died on October 2, 2015, seven months after the release of the animal shelter report. Keith Jackson, with whom I had not spoken since that day I entered his place of business, in tears, carrying that 464-page report, in a text to me asked if it would be okay if he attended her funeral.

"Of course, it would be," I replied.

CHAPTER 59

State Report: Lawton Pound Sucks but More Importantly, Facebook Sucks Worse — Posted by YesBiscuit

ON MARCH 23, 2015, internet blogger Yes Biscuit, who obviously had never been to Lawton in his or her life, saw the report for what it was and posted the following:

"The Oklahoma State Board of Veterinary Medical Examiners conducted an investigation into allegations of neglect and other wrongdoing at the Lawton pound at the request of the city manager. The 464 page report starts out with a page titled 'Conspiracy and Connection of Defendants.' On one side of the chart featured on this page is a local spay-neuter clinic and on the other side is a Facebook page with various uh, conspirators named below each. Yes, that says Facebook Page.

"The Facebook page is administered by a group called Lawton Citizens for Humane Treatment of Animals. On that page, which I have not visited, people apparently post complaints regarding the mistreatment and killing of animals at the Lawton pound. I know this because the board's lead investigator has screencapped a ton of inflammatory posts from that page and included them in the report. To show that some people act like dicks on Facebook, I guess.

"If you are interested in reading a bunch of trash talk and the investigator's wagging-finger-o- shame responses, knock yourself out. The gist of the report, in my interpretation, is that oh sure, animals were being neglected and starved to death at the Lawton pound but you know, Facebook is terribleawfulsuperblech. And the employees are doing the best they can.

"Here are a few items I fished out of the muck and summarized that don't have anything to do with Facebook:

"Page 27, Item 69: Employees complained to the investigator that neither the kennel staff nor the ACOs had been properly trained; kennel staff refused to do their jobs and refused to follow instructions from supervisors; male staff refused to wash bowls or do laundry because it's 'woman's work'; sick and injured animals were left to suffer without veterinary care. "Page 28, Item 70 and 72: If the rescue group trying to pull a pet was not liked by the employees, they would kill the animal in retaliation.

"Page 28, Item 73: A dog was placed in a kennel with a dog who was known to be a resource guarder so that workers wouldn't have to clean an additional cage. (This was reportedly not an uncommon practice.) The resource guarder prevented the other dog from eating and the dog starved to death after 3 weeks. One of the employees responsible for the dead dog's feeding and daily care has since been transferred to the Lawton police department.

"Recommendations, Pages 39 - 40:
! Rotate animal killing shifts among the entire staff so that each person gets a longer break between killing shifts.
! Ban all the people who talk smack on Facebook.
! Sharing information and photos from inside the facility should be "strictly prohibited.
! The city needs to re-evaluate the practice of allowing animals discovered to be pregnant during spay surgery to give birth.
! Staff should be trained in areas such as basic animal care.
! A fresh coat of paint!

"The city manager says that by July 1, all the violations noted in the report will be brought into compliance. I would note that one of those violations was starving a dog to death. But yeah, let's silence the critics, start killing unborn puppies and kittens, slop some paint on the place and call it good. The Oklahoma State Board of Veterinary Medical Examiners must be so proud."

CHAPTER 60

"I volunteered to certify Lawton Animal Shelter employees in proper euthanasia techniques in 1989 to 1991. The euthanasia room had no electrical outlet so hair could not be shaved where it was needed over a vein. This required an even higher level of employee proficiency. After about two years of this, I could not force myself to continue the certification. The piles of dead animals there still haunt me." — Dr. Kenneth Reynolds, DVM, MPH, Animal Birth Control Clinic veterinarian

ON MAY 17, 2015, on the occasion of the thirtieth anniversary of the clinic and two months after the report had been released in March, we placed a full-page ad in the local newspaper, the same newspaper that had made the release of the report its front-page feature story—complete with its erroneous and libelous content—on Friday, March 20th, the day after the report was released and again, two days later, in their Sunday edition on March 22nd.

Our ad was entitled Celebrating 30 Years With Integrity! A History of the Animal Birth Control Clinic. (Notice we underlined the words with integrity). It was time that Lawtonians learned the real story about the Animal Birth Control Clinic and its 30-year struggle with the Oklahoma State Board of Veterinary Medical Examiners—as well as the Federal Trade Commission ruling against them—and all the other muck (that word is so appropriate, thank you YesBiscuit) set forth in G. Dale Fullerton's report. I affixed my byline to the ad.

Much of the contents of the ad was what I have already written in this book in that it was a condensed history of the Animal Birth Control Clinic as well as a condemnation of Fullerton's kill-the-messenger report. Following are excerpts from the lengthy ad:

"On May 23, 1985, The Animal Birth Control Clinic, one of the earliest high-volume, low-cost spay clinics in the nation, opened its doors to a waiting list of more than 100 pet owners in desperate need of low-cost neuters and spays.

"Six months earlier, a small group of Lawton citizens had met to discuss the overwhelming problem of stray dogs and cats on Lawton streets and county roads . . .

"Several of us at that meeting live in the county and were, ourselves, plagued with unmanageable numbers of abandoned dogs and cats. We all came to the same conclusion: We could not in a lifetime find homes for all the animals with which we were dealing. This organization would have to be dedicated to problem-solving, which meant reducing the number of unwanted dogs and cats. That could only be accomplished by massive, affordable neuters and spays.

"Six months later, the Animal Birth Control Clinic arose from the ashes of our attempts to involve local veterinarians in a community-wide neuter/spay effort.

"Struggling with the financial challenges of a low-cost spay clinic—which we subsidized with garage sales and other fund-raising events—was the easy part. What we hadn't anticipated was the unrelenting opposition we would face from local veterinarians and the Oklahoma State Board of Veterinary Medical Examiners . . .

"On July 2, 1986, a headline appeared in this newspaper that read: "Animal clinic temporarily closed." . . . That was news to us. The clinic was indeed open and twenty dogs and cats were sitting in their cages waiting for surgery the next day.

"A retraction appeared the next day on July 3, 1986 . . .

"We didn't miss a beat. We never have.

"Green's (writer of the article) articles quoted from the Oklahoma Veterinary Practice Act's Rules of Professional Conduct . . .

"Dr. Michael Benham, then secretary of the OSBVME said 'enforcement of the law is not an attempt to suppress competition between veterinarians and such low-cost clinics but is aimed at protecting the integrity of veterinarians and veterinary medicine.'

"The Federal Trade Commission didn't see it that way!

"In the spring of 1988, I surprisingly, received a call from Kristin Malmberg with the Dallas Regional Office of the Federal Trade Commission. Ms. Malmberg was seeking information regarding the contentious relationship between the OSBVME and the Animal Birth Control Clinic . . .

"On September 26, 1989, Ms. Malmberg faxed me a copy of a Federal Trade Commission press release with headlines that read: 'FTC CHARGES OKLAHOMA STATE VETERINARY BOARD ILLEGALLY RESTRICTED COMPETITION: BOARD AGREES TO SETTLE CHARGES.'

"The ruling can be read online and holds sway today . . .

"How could we have possibly guessed that in 2015, the Oklahoma State Board of Veterinary Medical Examiners would, once again, enter into our lives in such an ugly, life-changing, integrity-impugning manner?

"On learning who the city had requested to conduct the recent animal shelter investigation, we immediately called Councilman Keith Jackson to protest, insisting that the investigator had an indisputable conflict of interest. Unfortunately, our concerns fell on deaf ears at city hall. Considering the history and the glaring conflict of interest that existed, it was predictable that investigator G. Dale Fullerton of the Oklahoma State Board of Veterinary Medical Examiners would turn what should have been an unbiased investigation of the animal shelter into an indictment of the Animal Birth Control Clinic, and anyone associated with it.

"Fullerton's report is inundated with half-truths, innuendoes and downright lies. The fact that a dog starved to death at the animal shelter—let me repeat that—a dog starved to death!—obviously in the mind of the investigator, paled in significance to the fact that a Clinic employee spoke on KSWO TV; or that the clinic didn't keep records on animals it never treated.

"The fact that 196 animals, by the city's own statistics, were found dead in their cages or pens (that's one every other day!) was not as important to the investigator as the fact that Beverly Perry reported the number at over 200— a minor discrepancy. (Note: It would later be learned the actual documented number was 205).

"Incidentally, at that time we had only recently met Ms. Perry, even though Fullerton listed us as 'close personal friends' in his diagram labeled 'Conspiracy and connection of defendants.'

"The investigator took clinic employee Susan Barmettler and I to task for estimating the number of animals seen each week at the ABC Clinic. Fullerton reported that Barmettler claimed the clinic sees over 100 pets a week, while I reported we see more than 150 pets a week. "Documented clinic records reveal that during the week of March 2, the clinic saw 175 animals; for the week of March 9, it was 231; the week of March 16 was 258; and for the last week of March the figure was 183—proof positive that neither I nor Ms Barmettler overstated the facts! And, by the way, what did any of this have to do with an investigation of the Lawton Animal Shelter?

"The creation of two Facebook sites...obviously irked the investigator, and citizen complaints were, for the most part ignored—if not ridiculed!

"Space here does not permit revelation of the astonishing number of inaccuracies in G. Dale Fullerton's report. It doesn't take a mental giant, however, to recognize that it is slanted and unprofessional. A national blogger, who has never even been to Lawton, read the report and saw it for what it was.

"The question to City Hall and to G. Dale Fullerton is this: What is different about animal welfare activists speaking out in 2014 than it was in 1986? Have our Freedom of Speech rights changed since then? Did we miss something? The same activists who established the ABC Clinic formed the Humane Society solely to contract with the city to operate the then-deplorable animal shelter that was a stepchild of the Lawton Police Department.

"Without the Internet or cell phones, we found a way to be heard. We bought newspaper ads and wrote letters to the editor. We attended council meetings—and spoke there multiple times. And, yes, we circulated petitions at the Animal Birth Control Clinic, and elsewhere. We've circulated multiple petitions over the years—without retaliation. In America, we have a word for that. It's called Democracy!

On a hot Sunday afternoon in August, armed with a permit and led by former Councilman Bob Shanklin, we marched in protest at the shelter where animals were locked in a tin-roofed building with no ventilation; where rain poured in by the bucketfuls; and rats, the size of small kittens, called the place home. We were exercising our right to assemble and protest!

"We had been anything but silent when two animal control officers were fired because they allowed a cocker spaniel to die a cruel death, locked in a detached garage in Old Town North . . .

"No one objected when we brought in shelter experts Phyllis Wright and Bernie Weller with the Humane Society of the United States; Jennifer Orme with American Humane Association; Dr. Alice DeGroot, retired Albuquerque veterinarian and national shelter consultant. We even called PETA to intervene in a greyhound cruelty case involving a city employee.

"On June 4, 1986, Barbara Cassidy, Director of Animal Sheltering with HSUS, wrote a letter to City Manager Robert Metzinger in support of us, as did State Senator Billie Floyd of Ada, and John Hatchel, Deputy City Manager of Waco, Texas. Patrick Parkes, Vice-President of Field Services of the Humane Society of the United States wrote a letter of commendation for the work of the ABC Clinic in the battle against pet overpopulation. This is only a minuscule list of experts who weighed in on animal problems in our community.

"If animal activism galls G. Dale Fullerton and current city officials, one can only imagine what an investigative report would have looked like back in those days!

"There is no doubt we annoyed some people back then. Activists always do! However, we did all those things—exercising our Freedom of Speech rights—without anyone naming us as 'defendants' or accusing us of 'conspiring to damage Lawton Animal Welfare and its employees;' or 'demonstrating conduct that did deceive and harm the public;' or recommending we be banned from the Lawton Animal Shelter.

"Advocating for animals is not a crime and those of us who do that hardly deserve to have our names dragged through the mud!

G. Dale Fullerton states in his report that the OSBVME wants us, the defendants, to reimburse them the total cost of this investigation! Is this right out of the twilight zone or what?

"In spite of uncontrollable tears mixed with anger, shock, bewilderment, embarrassment and disbelief, as well as irreparable damage to our reputations by G. Dale Fullerton's slanted and slanderous report, the Animal Birth Control Clinic remains strong. The publicity has inspired more and more pet owners to responsibly have their pets fixed; and customers are sympathetic and supportive.

"The welfare of the animals, after all, is what it's all about. It's what it's always been about. For thirty years we've fought—with integrity, in spite of what G. Dale Fullerton would have you believe—for the humane treatment of animals. Animal cruelty, like child abuse, is everyone's business, and we must not allow bullying or intimidation to prevent us from speaking out for those who cannot speak for themselves!

"There's much to be done. Although critical to the cause, neutering and spaying and adoptions are, unfortunately, not solving the pet overpopulation problem. It's imperative that we ramp up the dialogue about the ultimate and indisputable culprit that causes pet overpopulation—and continue to press for laws that restrict pet breeding all across the nation.

In 1990, Dr. G. Gordon Robinson, then director of the Bergh Memorial Animal Hospital in New York, wrote an article entitled 'How to Keep a Humane Society Hospital out of your Community,' in which he explained the historical clash between spay clinics and veterinarians. He conceded that animal advocates 'don't look at it as getting into the surgery business; they look at it as getting out of the killing business.

"We are grateful, from the bottom of our hearts, for courageous veterinarians across the country, who risk harassment from their medical boards to work for humane organizations and perform high-volume, low-cost neuters and spays. They get it! They understand we want out of the killing business!

"Thank you, thank you, thank you to all who have supported us and believed in us throughout the years—and especially so in this most recent difficult time."

Inasmuch as we are a member of the Lawton Chamber of Commerce, they joined with us to host an open house at the Clinic on Friday, May 22, 2015, two months after the release of the now infamous animal shelter report conducted by an employee of the Oklahoma State Board of Veterinary Medical Examiners at the request of the supervisor of the Lawton Animal Shelter herself.

CHAPTER 61

"In keeping silent about evil, in burying it so deep within us that
no sign of it appears on the surface, we are implanting it, and it will
rise up a thousand fold in the future. When we neither punish nor
reproach evildoers, we are not simply protecting their trivial old age,
we are thereby ripping the foundations of justice from beneath new
generations." — Aleksandr Solzhenitsyn, Russian Author

THIS BOOK HAS been in the making for five years—perhaps six or even
more. I have had very little interest in revisiting it in the years since the death
of my daughter and the release of the animal shelter report. There is no way in
which I can explain, categorize, or even make sense of a report so dishonest in its
content as to render it immoral and without an ounce of credibility. Were I to
attempt that, this book, no doubt, would never be finished.

Therefore, I am not even going to attempt to do that. The 464-page report is
on the Internet where it will, most likely, remain for eternity, with all its criticisms
of Linda and I, as well as our employees at the Animal Birth Control Clinic, and
the many other compassionate citizens of this community—with very little or
no criticism of those who perpetuated the indescribable inhumane treatment
of animals and other wrongdoing at the Lawton Animal Shelter. The reader of
this book is welcome to, in the words of YesBiscuit "knock yourself out" reading
the "trash talk" and the "investigator's wagging-finger-o-shame responses" and
make up your own mind as to who is telling the truth: Those who starved a dog
to death or those of us who were horrified by the fact that a dog was starved
to death—in a tax-supported animal shelter with a budget of $750,000 and a
recently finished building for the needs and comfort of the supervisor and the
part-time veterinarian!

STILL UNABLE TO cope with our disbelief of the injustices associated with
the shelter and the dishonesty of the shelter report, on December 20, 2015, once
again we placed a large ad in the newspaper. Somehow, we had to find a way to
tell our story and how we had been wronged. We positioned the ad as an open
letter to those within the city government who had allowed such an erroneous
and libelous report to be released to the public.

This ad is also lengthy and sometimes repetitive to other sections of this book, but, is once again an attempt to give you an encapsulated version of the 464-page report.

The headline of the ad read: SHAME ON YOU, CITY OF LAWTON: An Open Letter to Mayor Fitch, City Manager Ihler, Assistant Manager Russell and Members of the Lawton City Council. I once again penned the ad and added, at the end, that it was supported by Linda Reinwand, Pascall Osborne, Susan Barmettler, Beverly Perry, Linda Wilson and Cathy Aycock. Again, some of it is repetitive, however, it provides additional insight into the seriousness of the attack on Lawton citizens. Excerpts from the ad are as follows:

"It was March 19, 2015,when you, the leaders of the City of Lawton, allowed the release of G. Dale Fullerton's report of the investigation of the Lawton Animal Shelter.

"What sort of thinking, or lack thereof, did it take for you to allow innocent citizens to become victims of what one local attorney described as a 'hatchet job?' . . .

"I knew from the outset that this investigator had a serious conflict of interest in several areas, but mainly with the Animal Birth Control Clinic due to a Federal Trade Commission ruling against Oklahoma veterinarians with regard to the legality of a non-profit operating a low-cost spay clinic.

"I had predicted a report that would put the clinic in a bad light, and I had shared those concerns with some of you. But what I was seeing in this report was mind boggling . . .

"Considering Fullerton's several conflicts of interest and his 'hatchet job' report, one has to wonder if the real conspiracy was shelter associates and Fullerton, and perhaps you, City leaders, actually conspiring against citizens . . .

"I was labeled as one of the 'defendants.' So was Animal Birth Control Clinic volunteer Administrator Linda Reinwand, as well as two clinic employees, Susan Barmettler and Pascall Osborne.

"Beverly Perry, creator of Lawton Citizens for the Humane Treatment of Animals Facebook (LCHTA) page was also listed as a defendant, along with her mother Linda Wilson and her sister Cathy Aycock. A box in the middle of the diagram connected us at the ABC Clinic with Perry, Wilson, and Aycock and called us 'Close Personal Friends,' even though most of us had just recently met.

"Actually, Perry had been contacted early on by General Lee Baxter (Ret.) who was expressing a desire to join the campaign, and in more than one meeting with him, Perry was advised to keep her distance from us at the ABC Clinic, due to our historic outspoken animal activism, which she did. None of us at the clinic had ever seen or had any input whatsoever into the slide presentation or notebook she presented to you at a later city council meeting. Perry was in what was referred to as the Baxter and Phyllis Robertson 'camp' and we were described as the ABC Clinic 'camp.' How your investigator turned that into a conspiracy, and why you allowed a report that alleged such a conspiracy to be released, is beyond logical comprehension and leaves us guessing as to the motive.

"Baxter and Humane Society President Robertson and her organization magically escaped the investigator's wrath in the report, even though it was Robertson who had distributed the kennel worker's now famous letter of discontent to the ABC Clinic—which was, in large part, what set off a shelter investigation in the first place. It was also humane society fosters who were reporting many of the concerns at the animal shelter . . .

"Ironically, my role in all of this was very limited. My daughter's cancer was beginning to take a downward spiral around that time. I remember telling Councilwoman Rosemary Bellino, in a phone conversation, that I didn't want this to be happening; that I was saddened by all of this, but that there were just too many complaints for it to be ignored, and that I could have only a very limited role of involvement because my daughter was my first priority.

"I don't believe I had yet met Beverly Perry at that time. But I thank God for her diligence in undertaking the task of bringing most of the citizen complaints to light. Ms. Reinwand and I have been concerned for years about the need for a young fearless voice for animals in this community. I have the greatest respect for anyone who has the guts to speak out for those who cannot speak for themselves.

"Many of us have contributed untold hours of volunteer labor and personal financial resources to the animal welfare cause in this community for more than three decades. There is no doubt the high volume neuters and spays at the ABC Clinic have reduced the numbers of animals handled each year by the City thus saving millions in tax dollars over those years. Have we ever asked for anything in return or even a simple thank you? No! And that's not important. But do we deserve to be labeled liars, accused of using 'false, fraudulent, and deceptive statements?' and 'demonstrating conduct that did deceive and harm the public?' Ruth Steinberger, who introduced and promoted calcium chloride castrations at the shelter, wrote on *the Lawton Constitution* Facebook page that we might be 'people creating turmoil for fun or retribution?'

"Do you really believe we are thieves who stole shelter veterinary records as your investigator implied? How would we even have done that? Do you really believe, as your investigator inferred, that Ms. Perry never held the position of Global Head of Device Safety Operations in Research and Development with the largest pharmaceutical-medical device company in the world, where she worked in over 50 countries for that company for 17 years? And could just one of you explain to any of us what Ms. Perry's professional career had to do with an investigation of the Lawton Animal Shelter anyway? Was this your investigator's attempt to belittle and embarrass her as he attempted to do to the rest of us? Or was this perhaps retaliation for her refusal to take down her Facebook page as some of you demanded?

"The one thing we know for sure, City of Lawton leaders, is that this report was allowed to be released by you, and we believe you knew sections of the report were completely false. It should have been obvious to you in your closed-door executive session that this report was not credible—that it was primarily targeting citizens. But not one of you stood up publicly for the truth. Not one! No one even quietly said to any of us that you disagreed with the report. You allowed the 'hatchet job' to reach public view in not one, but two days of front page reporting in this newspaper, as well as on TV and the internet, where it will remain accessible to the world throughout eternity. Bryan Long told the media it was a 'quality' report.

"Ms. Perry's name was listed 101 times, with 23 additional references to 'she' or 'her,' in the 37-page report, not including attachments. I haven't had the stomach to count how many times the ABC Clinic and those of us connected to it were listed, but it was far more often than your name was listed, Mr. Ihler, where the 'buck' should have stopped. In fact, your name rarely appeared in the report and Supervisor Rose Wilson's was listed only minimally in comparison.

"This report has damaged us in ways you, City of Lawton leaders, are obviously incapable of understanding—far beyond hurt feelings, outrage, defamation of character and violation of our First Amendment rights. Do you know how difficult it is to face business associates, your doctors, your daughter's doctors, newly-made acquaintances, even funeral directors, and others, knowing they read the newspaper and watch TV? Our only comfort is knowing truth is on our side. "Your willingness, City of Lawton leaders, to release a report so devoid of substantial credibility has made us distrust our city government, and question just what could possibly be behind all this. You knew there were problems at the shelter. Citizens were coming out of the proverbial woodwork with horror stories. You knew that dogs had died from starvation, and from complications associated with calcium chloride castration, by your own admission, Mr. Ihler. It was discussed openly at a meeting where some of us were present, as well as some council members and former City Manager Bryan Long. Those deaths were mentioned in the kennel worker's original letter, however, that one sentence was mysteriously absent from Ms. Wilson's response.

"You knew that dogs and cats were found dead in cages every other day. You knew that seriously injured dogs and cats were allowed to suffer for days without medical care, or even humane euthanasia. Perry had provided information, including photographs and medical records of citizen complaints, all of which were given little attention by your investigator, or never even investigated at all. He was obviously preoccupied with investigating us.

"Why didn't you just 'own' the problems at the shelter, make some needed changes, make truth and transparency standard operating procedure, and move ahead? Why did you decide, instead, to allow a 'hatchet job' on innocent citizens?

"Two lawsuits are already in process. Some of us may not go that route, but all of us—citizens who have been deeply wronged—will speak out to clear our names in the court of public opinion. You, City of Lawton leaders, may find it necessary to, once again, huddle behind closed doors in one of your private executive sessions to discuss just what should be done about us.

"Make no mistake. This has nothing to do with revenge. We simply must not allow these injustices heaped upon innocent citizens to go unchecked, 'thereby ripping the foundations of justice from beneath new generations.'

"Dogs and cats suffered and died, and people lied, and the one thing you can count on is this: We will not be silenced!"

CHAPTER 62

"Animals don't have a voice, but I do. A loud one. A big f***ing mouth. My voice is for them. And I'll never shut up while they suffer." — Ricky Gervais, actor and comedian

AS THIS BOOK nears completion, I have toyed with the idea of changing the name wherein I omit Veterinarians, Humane Societies and Others Against Animals, and simply call the book *The Politics Behind the Killing of America's Pets.*

And then I learn of a recent Washington Post online article written in April, 2018, entitled "Dog Fight—Dog Rescuers, flush with donations, buy animals from the breeders they scorn."

The headline was troublesome enough, but what I read within the article written by Kim Kavin enraged and sickened me.

"An effort that animal rescuers began more than a decade ago to buy dogs from $5 or $10 apiece from commercial breeders has become a nationwide shadow market that today sees some rescuers, fueled by Internet fundraising, paying breeders $5,000 or more for a single dog," wrote Kavin.

"The result is a river of rescue donations flowing from avowed dog saviors to the breeders, two groups that have long disparaged each other. The rescuers call many breeders heartless operators of inhumane "puppy mills" and work to ban the sale of their dogs in brick-and-mortar pet stores. The breeders call 'retail rescuers' hypocritical dilettantes who hide behind nonprofit status while doing business as unregulated, online pet stores," the article stated.

I never would have believed that I would agree with breeders on anything, however, they have it right in their description of the "hypocritical dilettantes."

According to Kavin's article, for years the rescuers have come together with breeders at these dog auctions and some breeders contend that more puppies are being bred to sell to the rescuers.

The article says that bidders affiliated with "86 rescue and advocacy groups and shelters throughout the United States and Canada have spent $2.68 million buying 5,761 dogs and puppies from breeders since 2009 at the nation's two government-regulated dog auctions, both in Missouri, according to invoices, checks and other documents The Washington Post obtained from an industry insider."

Obviously, the rescuers offer the dogs for adoption as "rescued" or "saved."

My God! Is there anything humans haven't thought of, or done, to exploit man's best friend! "Most of the breeders who sell dogs at auction are commercial, which means they have at least four breeding females, sell to intermediaries and are federally regulated," wrote Kavin.

Regulated, yes, but enforced? Probably not. Does regulated breeding ever mean restricted or limited breeding except in communities with strict mandatory neuter/spay laws? Doubtful. According to the article, rescuers maintain that the "success of the rescue movement in reducing shelter populations has been driving rescuers to the auction market."

"As the number of commercial kennels has decreased," wrote Kavin "so has the number of shelter animals killed in the United States: A February 2017 estimate put the total for dogs alone at 780,000, a steep drop from estimates for all shelter animals that were as high as 20 million in the 1970s."

I have no expertise in the estimated numbers of shelter animals being tossed around in recent years and I pay little attention to those who claim they do. Frankly, I don't believe that anyone has an accurate number.

Perhaps we should revisit an earlier chapter in this book wherein nationally-known animal advocate Ed Duvin in his articles "Benign Neglect" and "In the Name of Mercy" took the shelter establishment to task for record keeping and the "shameful non-existence of national shelter statistics. Although shelters have existed in this country for well over a century, there is simply no reliable statistical base from which even the most basic information can be derived," he wrote.

I personally am convinced that there is still no accurate record keeping in American animal shelters on a national level today. As I have written earlier, there is no county animal control in vast parts of this country, certainly not in Oklahoma. Common sense dictates that no one in Podunk America is keeping track of how many dogs and cats are homeless in their neck of the woods and, even if they were, they are not being shared with any organizations that are gathering statistics.

I am going to repeat what I wrote in another chapter, and I believe it with my entire being: No matter what website you visit, or who you speak to, everyone has a different number for animal killings in American shelters—simply because no one knows for sure!

In fairness, I would concede that shelter numbers are most likely lower than in previous years due to the no-kill push for shelter adoptions as opposed to purchasing puppies and kittens but more likely due to the increasing nationwide emphasis on neutering and spaying, as well as the availability, in many communities, of low-cost sterilizations.

Some time ago, Nathan Winograd, leader of the no-kill movement, posted a suggestion that perhaps a TNR (Trap, Neuter, Release) program, which deals with feral cats, should be started for dogs.

My friend Beverly responded to his wacky idea by telling him he just disproved his theory. "If there is no pet overpopulation problem why do you need programs to deal with stray dogs." Actually, in a no-kill world, why would we even need a Trap, Neuter, Release program for cats?

I hasten to add that there are kind, compassionate and loving people caring for animals in the no-kill movement. I just cannot see how adoptions or buying dogs from breeders at auctions can end pet overpopulation without restrictions on pet breeding. The math won't work!

The thirty-three page Washington Post article can be read online. If one is interested, and can somehow stomach the information contained therein, as my new unknown friend, YesBiscuit would say "Knock yourself out."

With friends like these, dogs damn sure don't need enemies!

And no, no. Hell no. I won't change the title of this book!

I wonder what property in Alta, Utah is going for now.

Although this is her first book, Deloris Delluomo has been a prolific writer for most of her adult life. She published *Lawton Magazine*, which later expanded to *Texhoma Monthly*, and *The Lawton Times*, a small weekly newspaper, in which she wrote feature articles, two of the most notable being interviews with country music star Hank Williams, Jr., and Larry Jones of the International charity Feed the Children. She has written op-ed pieces for *The Lawton Constitution, The Daily Oklahoman*, and *The Oklahoma Observer*.

Although she was born and raised in rural Oklahoma, she has lived in Cleveland, Kansas City, and Phoenix, and traveled the world with her late husband in his capacity as a Nissan automobile dealer from 1975 to 1995.

She and her husband raised four children. Dana, Monty, Jamie, and Paul, all of whom have been or are serious animal advocates. Two children, Melissa Ann and Chris Michael, died shortly after birth. She lives in Lawton, OK.

www.ingramcontent.com/pod-product-compliance
Lightning Source LLC
Chambersburg PA
CBHW031501270326
41930CB00006B/192